PATIENTS, POWER & POLITICS

D1189455

PATIENTS, POWER & POLITICS

From Patients to Citizens

CHRISTINE HOGG

SAGE Publications
London • Thousand Oaks • NewDelhi

First published 1999

SAGE Publications Ltd
6 Bonhill Street
London EC2A 4PU

SAGE Publications Inc
2455 Teller Road
Thousand Oaks, California 91320

SAGE Publications India Pvt Ltd
32, M-Block Market
Greater Kailash – I
New Delhi 110 048

British Library Cataloguing in Publication Data

A catalogue record for this book is
available from the British Library

ISBN 0 7619 5877 0
ISBN 0 7619 5878 9 (pbk)

Library of Congress catalog record available

Typeset by Keystroke, Jacaranda Lodge, Wolverhampton.
Printed in Great Britain by Athenaeum Press, Gateshead

CONTENTS

To my parents, who showed me the value of being
a non-conformist

ACKNOWLEDGEMENTS

Many people have helped me in writing this book, by their encouragement, sharing their experiences and commenting on drafts. I would like to give special thanks to Eileen O'Keefe whose enthusiasm encouraged me to start out. I would also like to thank Frances D'Souza, the people of Capileira and the Universidad for making writing it such fun.

Many people have read drafts and given me their comments in particular Melanie Fennell, Eileen Lepine, Robert Maycock, Naomi Pfeffer and Gill Tremlett. I would also like to thank Beverley Lawrence Beech, Stephen Fuller, David Gilbert, Sally Hogg, Muriel Hogg, Sophie Laws, Gill Procter, Anne Rivett, Jean Robinson, Mai Wann, Charlotte Williamson, Fedelma Winkler and Jack Winkler.

1

INTRODUCTION

Patients, of course, have roles assigned to them within the scripts of the modern medical drama. Depending on who is doing the analysis or the accountancy, patients appear as demand, costs and benefits, input or output, voters, clients or consumers of services, bearers of rights or pursuers of litigation, the 'tib' and 'fib' in bed 15, frozen sperm in the deep freeze, diseased bodies or clinical material, points on a graph or numbers crunched on a software programme.

Roy Porter, *Greatest Benefit to Mankind* (1997)

History is written by the victors. What we know about English history after 1066 relied on the versions written or sponsored by the French conquerors. Until recently the history of America, Australia and Africa was the history of the white settlers. There is an alternative story, generally suppressed: the story of the English under the Normans and of the native Americans, Australians and Africans.

Similarly, the analysis of current health issues is based on the experiences of people who are in a position to get their views heard: politicians, clinicians, managers, economists and drug companies. Political debates and decisions on health policy are based on their analyses of the problems and the negotiations, disputes and alliances between them. In 1997 the White Paper, *The New NHS – Modern, Dependable NHS*, stated: 'decisions about how to best use resources for patient care are best made by those who treat patients – and this principle is at the heart of the proposals' (Department of Health, 1997b: 7). Certainly, people who provide services need to be involved in making decisions, but so do the people affected by these decisions – health service users. The interests of the public and users of health care are evoked to support particular interests in these negotiations, sometimes by professionals, sometimes by managers and sometimes by the pharmaceutical companies. Health care professionals, managers and pharmaceutical companies appeal to the public to support them to achieve the health care system they are aiming for. Doctors argue for their clinical freedom to do their best for patients and for more resources for their services. Managers talk of rationalizing services based on local needs, patient satisfaction and consulting with users – even of 'controlling' patient expectations. Meanwhile drug companies, who have for a long time targeted professionals to increase their sales, now target the public directly in order to raise their expectations and create consumer demand for their products. However, the public, as citizens or as users, have rarely been directly involved, except where their views coincide with those of the more powerful.

There are major upheavals going on in how health care is provided, and more and more is expected of health service users and those who represent their interests. Changes in the relative position of health service users have been rapid – after all, until the Medicines Act was passed in 1968 patients did not have the right to know the names of drugs prescribed for them. Not surprising then that there is confusion over the appropriate role for people who use health services. There is no word that everyone may comfortably use to describe the individual receiver of health or social care. Patient, client, customer, consumer and user are all used and each has different implications. The word 'patient' implies a compliance and passivity that reflects but also reinforces the unequal power between patient and professional; it also excludes carers, people who may use health services in the future and recipients of social care, normally called 'clients'. 'Consumer' or 'customer' is often used as this fits in with the business ethos that has been introduced into health care, but people receiving health care do not see themselves as consumers or customers and rarely have the choice that this implies. 'User' is a wider term that can include patients, potential patients, clients and carers, but it does not reflect the intimacy of the relationship that often exists between the receiver and giver of care or the unequal power balance between them. In this book individuals receiving health care are called 'patients', while the term 'user' includes everyone who uses or may use services in future, either as patients or carers.

This book looks at health care and public health from the perspective of users and citizens. 'Patients' have traditionally been expected to rely on experts for advice and be 'compliant'. However, the imbalance in the relationship between the patient and clinician raises basic ethical issues. Professionals have used incentives and sanctions to encourage people to comply with treatment, when they consider it to be in their 'best interests' or those of society. There have been changes, with patients being encouraged to see themselves as consumers with rights and, more recently, as 'partners' with responsibilities as well. However, there are still tensions and contradictions in the professional–patient relationship between paternalism and the individual's right to autonomy. There are problems in gaining access to independent information which would enable people to exercise their rights and responsibilities (Chapter 2).

The boundaries between health and illness are constantly shifting. Conditions previously seen as normal – such as being short, going through the menopause or even having a baby – have been redefined as 'problems' for medical science for which there are bio-medical solutions. In immunization and screening programmes, people are persuaded to use health services for which they may not see the need, either for their own good or for the public good. We cannot assume that we are healthy because we do not feel ill. Again there are tensions and conflicts between the individual's right to autonomy, the belief that the 'doctor knows best', and the good of society (Chapter 3).

Medicine is always looking forward hopefully, in search of better treatments and cures. Research policy is of great interest to the public since today's research determines the sort of treatments and services that will be available tomorrow. However, research is increasingly funded by pharmaceutical companies to meet their commercial needs. One result of this trend may be that studies provide evidence for the benefits but not the disadvantages of drugs and there will be little research into the effectiveness of other therapeutic approaches. Although research is carried out for the benefit of patients, they are generally excluded except as the subjects of research. Excluding users from research policy and design has meant that much health research is of poor quality and irrelevant to the experiences of patients and carers (Chapter 4).

While helping to strengthen the position of the individual user is important, there are many issues that can only be tackled by people as part of local communities and as citizens. Here again there is confusion about how users and citizens can contribute to health policy. At a local level, there is no democratic accountability in the health service. Though managers are expected to consult the public, it is up to individual managers how much notice they take of their views. However, there are some examples that show how even disadvantaged communities may be involved, using methods that empower them (Chapter 5).

Citizens elect governments which make policies that affect health. However, it is not generally possible to use votes to support particular health policies – they come with other policies as a job lot. Professionals, commercial interests and users each have different interests that some-times conflict and sometimes overlap. Though there may be alliances between all those interest groups, professional and commercial interests are in a better position to influence government since it needs their co-operation to implement policies. Voluntary organizations are, in comparison, poorly funded and unco-ordinated. Often funding depends on the alliances they make with professional and commercial interests and the support they give to government policies. Voluntary organizations are increasingly accepting sponsorship from commercial interests which may compromise their independence and ability to speak on behalf of users (Chapter 6).

National lobbying is no longer enough. More and more policies that affect health and the way that health services are organized are made by international bodies, such as the European Union, the World Health Organization, the World Bank and the World Trade Organization. Often decisions that affect health are made as part of negotiations about trade and tariffs, where health is a minor consideration. Commercial interests operate on a transnational level and it is important that there is a strong independent public interest and consumer movement to counterbalance commercial interests and to monitor their activities (Chapter 7).

In the midst of the upheavals in health services and public health, there is no clear vision of what we are trying to achieve. Current debates about rationing, scientific developments, regulation, audit, effectiveness and consumerism sometimes appear to be dominated by assumptions that need to be questioned. For example, people tend to assume that medicine is based in science and that any new technique or drug will be an improvement. In reality most health care is about chronic conditions that people live with for many years, and, in spite of greater scientific knowledge, diagnoses are uncertain and treatments unpredictable. Then there are newer assumptions that originate from an economist's view of health care: that demand for health care is infinite and that patients are consumers. In fact, 'demand' is created by professional and commercial interests as well as by patients. Furthermore, patients do not have the choice or information that is required to be true 'consumers' or even 'partners' (Chapter 8).

Developing health policy and health services that are user-centred requires action to strengthen the relative position of users and citizens at all levels. A user-centred health service would recognize that when people have health problems they do not just have clinical needs, but emotional, psychological, social and financial needs. The relationship between professionals and users would be rooted in respect for the autonomy of the individual. To achieve this, users need additional rights and responsibilities in the context of their position as citizens. They need access to independent information as well as advice to help them use this information effectively. Investment needs to be made to enable groups who represent users to participate as equals at national and international levels (Chapter 9).

In 1997 the government announced a ten-year plan for the NHS, emphasizing the importance of building partnerships with users, improving clinical effectiveness and governance, and addressing accountability. The test for this commitment will be whether users are allowed to speak for themselves in these changes or whether others will continue to speak for them.

PART I
THE INDIVIDUAL

2

PATIENTS

> Everyone who is born holds dual citizenship, in the kingdom of the well and in the kingdom of the sick. Although we all prefer to use only the good passport, sooner or later each of us is obliged, at least for a spell, to identify ourselves as citizens of the other place.
>
> Susan Sontag, *Illness as Metaphor*, (1991)

Everyone of us is at some time or another a patient. Most of the time we look after our own health, perhaps seeking information or advice from family and friends, magazines, or the pharmacist. Sometimes we have to ask for medical help and, when we do, we are 'patients' for the short time we are in contact with health services. Even then it is not primarily how we see ourselves. We are playing a role: the role of patient.

This chapter considers the changing, and often contradictory, expectations that underlie the rights and responsibilities of patients and professionals. There are different models that have been used to describe this relationship. In the traditional model of paternalism, professionals are deemed to know best and patients are required to trust them. Consumerism goes to the other extreme: individuals are in charge of getting the 'best buy' for their own health care and they cannot take the trustworthiness of professionals for granted. The partnership model sees the giving and receiving of health care as a negotiation agreed between the parties. Finally, there is the model of autonomy that puts respect for the individual first and recognizes the different perspectives of patients and professionals. Each model has its strengths and weaknesses for both users and professionals.

Who are 'patients'?

'Patients' are just people with particular health problems who may be taking medicines or receiving treatment. Generalizing about 'patients' can be misleading and ignore the great diversity in individuals' attitudes to health and expectations of health care. Patients and carers want different things from health services. Relationships with, and expectations of, health professionals will also be different according to who you are – education, social class, income, ethnic origin and lifestyle will all have influence on an individual's perspective. Some people, often because of barriers of language, race or disability, have problems in using health services and may receive a poor service.

At each stage in life people have a different attitude to health and want different things from health care. Babies and young children can become seriously sick very quickly, and until recently many babies and young children died in their first year. Children, particularly toddlers, are prone to accidents, especially where they live in poor housing and do not have safe areas to play and explore. Parents are often anxious about their children's health and make demands on health services.

Adolescence is a time of change and growing into an adult body is often disturbing and stressful. Young people may be concerned about their relationships, their physical appearance, their weight, puberty, acne and their sexuality. They are also more likely to take risks – such as experimenting with drugs, cars and motor cycles. Young people may be reluctant to talk about personal matters to a doctor who knows their family or use a service where staff seem judgemental.

Women are major users of health services. Women visit their GPs almost twice as often as men, consume more drugs and medicines than men, occupy acute hospital beds slightly more than men and are admitted to psychiatric units more than men (Kane, 1991). Having a baby used to be a risky business but it is now safer, both for mother and for baby. However, there is conflict between midwives, obstetricians and women about the best place to have a baby and the best way to manage labour; in particular, a stormy debate centres around how far nature should be allowed to run its course and when and how far professionals should intervene. Some writers from a feminist perspective see the way health care is provided to women as a way in which they are controlled and exploited (P. Foster, 1995).

Men are likely to die earlier than women. They are less likely to ask for help and, when they do, they are likely to be more seriously ill. Howard (1996) found that, when young, men felt that it was not 'macho' to fuss about their health; however, when they got older they were still reluctant to go to the doctor. Men had a low level of knowledge about male cancers, found it difficult to talk about health problems and were embarrassed by intimate examinations.

Finally, people are living longer, but with more disabling conditions and with a poorer quality of life. The extra years of life that have been achieved are extra years of disability, not of health (Dunnell, 1995).This puts demands on family and neighbours who look after older people. In old age people may live alone and be socially isolated; partners may have died and children moved away. Policies to develop primary health care and community care mean that people are now cared for in the community when before they would have been in hospital, whether as an in-patient after surgery or segregated in a large institution because of mental health problems.

At some point in our lives most of us are faced with the need to care for someone who is ill or disabled. Six million people in Britain take responsibility for the care of a friend or relative. Becoming a carer often leads to a reduction of income if you have to give up work. It may also mean being confined to the house if the person you look after cannot be left alone. The trend towards providing services in the community has meant that family and friends are under greater pressure to become carers. However, these pressures have coincided with other social trends such as more women working outside the home and having less time to care for elderly relatives, and more people living alone and choosing to do so.

Compliance and patients' responsibilities

By tradition, doctors are expected to be experts, adhere to high ethical standards and not to make mistakes. In return for their expertise and ethical standards, patients are expected to trust them and comply with their advice. Sir Raymond Hoffenberg puts the case for clinical freedom and paternalism:

> My concern to preserve the central role of the doctor in clinical decisions, moral or otherwise, is not a reflexion of professional self-interest or a wish to perpetuate professional sovereignty. It is based on my belief that such decisions must rest on a proper knowledge of all the medical consequences of each option, physical and psychological, qualitative as well as quantitative; that they must be made with critical and professional detachment; and that they should be conveyed to and discussed with the patient and the family with compassion and sensitivity. (1987: 72)

However, often people do not follow the instructions they are given or take their medicines as instructed. One in five patients do not even get as far as the pharmacy to collect the medicines that have been prescribed for them. Half of patients who suffer from chronic diseases do not take their medication in fully therapeutic doses (Royal Pharmaceutical Society of Great Britain, 1997). Sometimes there are serious consequences if you do not take medicines as instructed. For example, one study showed that 18 per cent of renal transplant patients did not follow instructions in taking their medication. Ninety-one per cent of these patients experienced organ rejection or died, while only 18 per cent of patients who adhered to the prescribed regimen experienced organ rejection or died (Rovelli et al., 1989). Non-compliance also means that side effects of drugs may be under-reported and research results may be based on inaccurate information.

From Compliance to Concordance, a report published in 1997 by the Royal Pharmaceutical Society of Great Britain, looked at how patients could be persuaded to take their medicines. It seemed to assume that patients had no rational reasons for non-compliance, but that their irrational reasons needed to be understood in order to deal with the problem:

> Researchers suggest . . . that the most salient and prevalent influences on medicine-taking are the beliefs that people hold about their medication and about medicine in general. These beliefs are often at variance with the best evidence from medical science and consequently receive scant, if any, attention from the prescriber. Yet they are firmly rooted in the personal and family and cultural experiences of us all. For the prescriber simply to reaffirm the views of medical science and to dismiss or ignore these beliefs, is to fail to prescribe effectively. (1997: 7)

The report was prepared by an advisory group of professionals, academics and representatives of a pharmaceutical company but had no representative of users or voluntary organizations.

However, there are many reasons why people do not take professional advice or look elsewhere for help and some of them are rational (Donovan and Blake, 1992). They may not admit that they are not following advice for fear of alienating professionals and being labelled as 'difficult'. Some people do not comply because of the nature of their illness, for example people with manic depression are most likely to stop taking medication as they move from depression to mania, which is when they need it. Some people may not collect medicines prescribed for them because they cannot afford the prescription charge or because they wanted some other kind of help when they went to the doctor.

Sometimes people do not take medicines because they perceive the cause of the problem and its solutions differently from professionals, such as people who are anxious and stressed but do not feel that drugs will help solve their problems. Some people who have received mental health care see themselves as passive recipients of coercive treatment and as survivors of the system, where intervention has created problems for them rather than helped them. A study found that mental health service users wanted a more active role in treatment and in planning services but that professionals found this threatening (Glenister, 1994). Many surveys have found that talking therapies, counselling and psychotherapy are rated more highly than other therapies. However, they were often not offered to people with severe conditions or to black and Asian people. People with mental health problems want more attention paid to helping them to manage their mental illness and to live with it. People find aromatherapy, art and creative therapies help them cope (Mental Health Foundation, 1997).

People may stop 'complying' when they find that orthodox medicine does not help them. Some people with chronic pain may feel like the 'failures' of modern medicine. They may see the whole range of specialists – orthopaedics, neurology, gynaecology, psychiatry and physical medicine – and receive many treatments, but still not get better. Orthodox services often only offer painkillers, which have side effects and become less and less effective over time. So people look for alternative ways of living with their pain. Some join self-help groups which provide opportunities to learn things from each other which can only be gained from people who have had the same or similar experiences.

For some patients, compliance with orthodoxy is the price they may have to pay for acceptance by professionals. If physical causes cannot be found for symptoms, the illness may be labelled 'psychosomatic' and the person transferred from mainstream medicine to psychiatry. People resent this if they feel that there is a physical cause for their illness. Some people may be considered to have adopted the 'sick role'. The 'sick role' is a concept developed by sociologist Talcott Parsons (1970). People occupying the sick role are not held responsible for their incapacity and are exempted from their usual obligations. However, in return, they must want to get well and seek and follow medical advice. If they do not behave in this way, they may lose the right to be thought of as sick. If they reject medical advice – based on their experience of what helps them – they may be dismissed as not really being as ill as they say they are. This can be very alienating and humiliating for people who do not fit easily into conventional diagnostic categories.

Though the language may change from 'compliance' to 'concordance', the pressures on patients may remain. Incentives for patients are generally seen as giving them better information and communicating with them better so that they understand the importance of following instructions. Sharing information may increase compliance but also, at times, may increase dissent. If people are aware of the risks they may not wish to take them, as, for example, seems to be the case in childhood immunization programmes (Chapter 3). Sometimes information is not enough and other incentives may be used where compliance is in the public interest. For example, if patients with tuberculosis (TB) do not comply with their medical treatment, they may pass the infection on to other people. In New York payment is made to encourage homeless people with TB to come for weekly treatments. Financial incentives are most likely to be effective for TB, antenatal and post-natal care, treatment for alcohol and drug abuse, and anti-rejection therapy and weight loss (Togerson and Giuffrida, 1997). There is, however, always the risk that people will take up the activity in order to qualify for the incentive to give it up; apparently some Russian prisoners deliberately infected themselves with TB in order to get into hospitals with better food and conditions.

Consent to treatment

When people seek medical help, this does not mean that they want to pass over all the responsibility to professionals, though they may want to share the responsibility. In all events, patients take the risks and have to live with the consequences of decisions about treatment. For many conditions diagnosis is often uncertain or the effects of treatment unpredictable. McPherson (1990) has argued that where this is the case, such as for prostate cancer, patients' preferences are very important in determining what treatment is given.

However, there is still some resistance to providing information to patients. In the past, when doctors had few effective medicines or treatments, they built up patients' confidence in their skills through magic. The power of magic depends on the audience not understanding how the effect is achieved: the audience does not need to know how the rabbit appears from the 'empty' hat. Clinicians relied on the placebo effect – that is, people's positive responses, at least initially, to almost any treatment as long as they believe in the treatment and trust the professional. The benefit may have nothing to do with the treatment itself and almost any treatment is as likely to be effective. When doctors relied on 'magic' for results, patients did not need information. From the mid-1950s doctors came to be seen more as scientists or technicians. For technical solutions, you also do not need to know how the part in your body (or your car) is repaired. You just need to know that it can be repaired. And so the resistance to sharing information has continued, though this is changing.

In 1991 the Patient's Charter gave people the right to have any proposed treatment, including any risks involved in that treatment and any alternatives, clearly explained to them before they decided whether to agree to it (Department of Health, 1991a). Consent has two different functions. One function is legal – without consent clinicians may be committing assault or trespass when they touch their patient. The idea that a person's bodily integrity should be protected from unauthorized touching or invasion has been part of English law since the Middle Ages. The second function is clinical and aims to secure the patient's trust and co-operation (Montgomery, 1997).

In spite of this, English law does not require that consent be fully informed. In general, the courts do not define patients' rights by what is adequate information to make a decision but by whether other reputable practitioners would have done the same. This was established in 1985 after Anne Sidaway was left partially paralysed as a result of an operation on her spine. This was not negligence but she sued because she was not told that the operation had a one to two per cent chance of causing paralysis. She lost the case because expert witnesses testified that some neurosurgeons would not have mentioned the risk of paralysis under similar circumstances. However, in the late 1990s the Senate of Surgery of

Great Britain and Ireland (1997) called for surgeons to go beyond what was legally required and give the information that a reasonable person would want to know.

The principle of informed consent recognizes that patients have the right to give their consent to treatment on the basis of full information. This was recognized as important in relation to research as part of the judgement at the Nuremberg trials after the Second World War and was later extended to clinical practice. Caroline Faulder (1985) has outlined five principles that underlie informed consent:

1 Autonomy – the individual's freedom to decide his or her own goals and to act according to those goals. This demands a respect for individuals even if the clinician disagrees with their views or actions.
2 Veracity – trust in doctors by patients must be based on truth and honesty.
3 Justice – both parties have a duty to treat each other justly, whether the doctor–patient relationship is seen as a contract, covenant or a partnership.
4 No harm – the doctor has a duty to do no harm.
5 Best interests – the doctor has a duty to act in the best interests of the patient.

The last two principles are used to justify refusing patients the right to give their informed consent. Each doctor has the duty to do what he or she sees to be in the best interests of the patient, even if the patient disagrees.

Overriding informed consent

Sometimes consent may be overridden. For example, the interests of research or teaching were at one time seen to override the right of patients to give informed consent, particularly where professionals do not see any harm in the procedure and consent might be refused. An example of this was allowing medical students to carry out internal vaginal examinations on women who were anaesthetized for an unrelated condition. The public were first made aware of this practice in November 1983 and were outraged. The practice was defended by medical schools as it was argued that this was the only way that medical students could get experience of internal examinations. This was, however, assault; and the implication was that the unconscious patient has less rights than a conscious person: if you are not aware that your rights have been infringed, it does not matter.

Some professionals are reluctant to accept the patient's right to refuse treatment because they believe that they know best. The doctor's duty to do 'good' is seen as more important than a patient's autonomy and rights over their own body. In the 1980s there were increasing numbers of interventions in maternity care ordered by the courts in the USA and, since 1992, in the UK. High Court hearings in obstetric cases do not always follow due process or comply with the principles of natural justice. Hearings are held in an emergency, and the women concerned are often not represented and may even be sedated at the time of the hearing. Even if they are represented, they may not have adequate opportunity to brief their advocate or obtain alternative clinical advice. The court is expected to make difficult judgements about the likely clinical outcome of an intervention, without adequate notice, in a clinical area where clinicians disagree about when intervention is necessary. In 1992 a High Court ruled that a woman should have a Caesarean section in order to protect the life of the foetus, though she had refused this on religious grounds. This was a curious ruling since it put the interests of the foetus before those of the woman, even though the foetus has no legal rights until it is born alive. In this case the Caesarean was performed but the baby died (Rock, 1995). In 1997 a Court of Appeal considered an emergency case of a woman with a needle phobia. After initially agreeing to a Caesarean, she changed her mind and refused when staff tried to give her an injection. She lost her case on the grounds that her needle phobia made her temporarily incompetent. However, the ruling upheld the woman's right to refuse intervention:

> The law is, in our judgement, clear that a competent woman who has the capacity to decide, may for religious reasons, other reasons, or for no reasons at all choose not to have medical intervention, even though, as we have already stated, the consequence may be the death or serious handicap of the child she bears or her own death. (Beech, 1997)

It remains to be seen if this is the last word.

Compliance with clinical treatment is seen as important for pregnant women to protect the health of the foetus. In some US states the foetus has rights; in other countries, as in the UK, the foetus only has rights when it is born alive. In the USA there are increasing numbers of prosecutions against women who have used drugs or alcohol during pregnancy which can result in babies being born addicted and needing to be withdrawn from drugs. Such attitudes may mean that some women try to avoid the health system, whereas, in fact, they need more antenatal care not less for their own and their baby's health. If drinking and using drugs in pregnancy are criminalized, what about damage caused by smoking or eating inadequate or inappropriate food? Criminalizing women with problems may deal with public anger, but it does not help the woman or baby.

In 1992 a 16-year-old girl with anorexia nervosa was made a ward of the court so that she could be force-fed to keep her alive. The High Court ruled that 16- and 17-year-olds have the right to consent to treatment, but not to refuse treatment, undermining established medical practice and the rights of young people. However, she could have been compulsorily treated under a section of the Mental Health Act 1983 (Hodgkin, 1993). In contrast, a court upheld the right of a man in Broadmoor Hospital with chronic schizophrenia to refuse to have his gangrenous foot amputated even though he was thought likely to die. The court determined that, though his mental capacity was impaired, it had not been established that he did not understand the purpose and effect of the treatment proposed (Montgomery, 1997). In the event he did not have his foot amputated, was treated with antibiotics and did not die.

Psychiatry has always been associated with social control as well as caring for or curing people with mental health problems. Until the end of the sixteenth century, people who were mentally ill were considered to be possessed by demons. Then mental illness gradually came to be regarded as a disease. As little could be done, mentally ill people were put away in lunatic asylums, which grew rapidly towards the end of the eighteenth century. The asylums were custodial and inmates had to be certified to be admitted. Later, fashionable views about eugenics and survival of the fittest led to inmates being ignored as degenerates. However, the First World War changed this. Large numbers of 'normal' middle-class men were 'shell-shocked' and their problems could not be dismissed as biological degeneracy or solved by segregating them from the rest of society. As a result the Tavistock Clinic was set up in 1920, with Field Marshal Haig and Admiral Beatty as vice presidents. However, the ascendancy of the asylums re-established itself as the direct aftermath of war passed. In the 1920s new treatments developed: insulin therapy, ECT (electro-convulsive therapy) and surgery on the frontal lobe of the brain (lobotomies). However, none of these were effective and they could lead to long-term damage. They were also used as a means of social control: women and people from disadvantaged communities were most likely to have a lobotomy or receive ECT (Breggin, 1993). In the 1950s tranquillizers were introduced, followed later by antidepressants. Many people were able to leave hospital and others were helped to cope at home rather than being admitted to hospital.

Sometimes the law and the Mental Health Act 1983 can be used to force patients to comply in their own 'best interest' (if they are thought to pose a risk to themselves), or to protect the public (if they are thought to pose a risk to others). This raises a genuine dilemma about the circumstances in which someone's right to make a decision should be respected, even if it means that they may die or there is a possibility, however slight, that they may harm others.

There can be long-term and damaging consequences of coercion for the individual. For example, anorexia nervosa mainly affects young people, mostly girls, who become obsessed with losing weight. At some point the weight loss becomes critical and their health – even their life – is put at risk. For many health service staff, the addiction to losing weight is incomprehensible and the solution is easy – to make the person eat. Staff experienced in working with eating disorders avoid coercion as far as possible as they are aware that the effects of re-feeding do not last. The individual may relapse and then be more resistant to treatment the next time. In a survey of people who had had eating disorders, of those people who had been admitted or detained against their wishes, 50 per cent said that they thought, in retrospect, it had been a 'good thing' (Newton et al., 1993).

Peter Breggin, an American psychiatrist, sums up the implications of the powers that psychiatrists have for mental health services: 'When we know we can use force to make people accept our "services", we have little motivation to offer better ones. If psychiatrists could not treat people against their will, they might try harder to develop something more appealing to potential consumers than drugs and electroshock' (1993: 468).

Children and young people

There are particular dilemmas in treating children. Legally children under 16 have the right to information and to be consulted about decisions that affect them according to their age and maturity. But how do you judge 'maturity'? Research by Priscilla Alderson (1990) has shown that children are often able to make informed and responsible decisions about their own health care and may have different views from their parents. Even very young children have views about their treatment and it is important for their well-being to involve them in decisions and help them feel that they are not powerless. When the father of Jaymee Bowen, aged 10, took legal action against the health authority which was refusing to fund a further bone marrow transplant to treat her leukaemia, she did not know that she was Child B in the sensational case that hit the headlines. When she found out, her comment was: 'Never give up. Because if you give up you will just end up with nothing left' (Barclay, 1996: 155). Towards the end of her life, as she suffered increasing difficulties, she was less certain about having further treatment and the fight for her life at all costs that her father was undertaking. 'If he arranges it behind my back, I would obviously be very upset. I'd feel really bad, but I want to be strong enough to refuse. Everyone has to die someday. Some earlier than others' (ibid.: 172).

Drugs given to children to control their behaviour highlight the potential conflict between the interests of parents and children. Parents tend to argue for physical causes for behaviour problems in their children and for medication to treat them, since this explanation relieves them of blame for what is happening to their child. Attention deficit hyperactivity disorders (ADHD) are seen as an increasing problem, especially among boys. This is a diagnosis that covers many forms of 'bad' behaviour, in particular an inability to concentrate which causes havoc at home and at school. Ritalin, an amphetamine, seems to work for some children and is prescribed to over one million children in the USA. It is increasingly prescribed in the UK, largely due to pressures from parent groups that have been set up to persuade doctors to prescribe it. There is little information about the long-term effects on children, but it is known that amphetamines are addictive in adults. Prescribing a drug may be cheaper and easier than attempting to understand the reasons for distressed behaviour, and devoting the time and resources to meet the special needs of difficult children in school and at home (Breggin, 1993).

Older children may not be willing to ask for advice on contraception, sexual health or substance use, if they believe that their parents are likely to find out. Assessing how far children under the age of 16 can give informed consent without the involvement of their parents is difficult. In 1986 Victoria Gillick took legal action against a health authority for giving contraceptive advice to girls under 16 without their parents' knowledge. The House of Lords, in giving judgement, emphasized that parental power to control a child exists not for the benefit of the parent but for the benefit of the child. Lord Scarman concluded: 'parental rights yield to the child's right to make his own decisions when he reaches a sufficient understanding and intelligence to be capable of making up his own mind on the matter requiring decision' (Montgomery, 1997).

People considered incapable

Where the patient cannot give informed consent, who should make the decision – for example, to withdraw life support systems? Under the law no one has the power to take decisions on medical treatment for an incapable adult. A relative's consent to treatment on behalf of an unconscious or incompetent adult is good practice but has no legal standing.

Ethics committees were set up in the USA in the 1980s to advise on withdrawing or withholding treatment when a patient is unable to give consent and are mandatory in some states. They were set up following the Karen Quinlan case in 1976. Karen Quinlan was a young woman in a coma on a life support system. Her parents won a court case against the hospital to get the life support system withdrawn. However, though the principle that a wider group should advise clinicians on difficult decisions seems sound, the actual practice is not proven. The best interest of the patient may not be the same as that of the hospital. The hospital may be primarily concerned to avoid litigation or the reallocation of resources. A review of US ethics committees found that many had tended to take advising the hospital as their primary role, rather than protecting patients (Hoffmann, 1993).

Some people with HIV who can anticipate their own deterioration and death have made 'living wills'. This allows them to maintain some control, even if they are no longer able to give instructions to professionals providing them with care. It is now recognized that if a patient in full command of his or her faculties refuses treatment, this should be respected, regardless of the patient's subsequent deterioration and incapacity (Doyle, 1997). The Law Commission recommended in 1995 that people should have the right to appoint friends or relatives to take medical decisions for them if they later become incapable. A Green Paper was published by the Lord Chancellor's Department in 1997 based on the Law Commission's report (Lord Chancellor's Department, 1997).

Sharing information

Respect for a person's autonomy and right to consent to or refuse treatment are central values in the relationship of clinician and patient. However, seeing clinical decisions in terms of informed consent may not be helpful in many consultations. Few decisions about health are 'now or never'. Most consultations and courses of treatment involve a series of choices, that lead from one to the next. There are options; you can try one and, if it does not work, try another. As the knowledge of both the clinician and the patient increases, it is possible to make more appropriate decisions.

The extent to which any individual patient wants to be involved will depend on the value they place on medical expertise. One study found that nearly half of patients asked wanted choice, but one fifth had reservations. One woman reported that she had written to the consultant: 'I said I appreciated being treated as an adult being able to make my own choices, yes I thought I was in control'; whereas another woman said: 'I thought it was the most traumatic thing. Why are you giving me this choice, you are the expert?' (Fallowfield, 1997).

Professionals may see information as less important than patients do (Nagel et al., 1992). Some professionals assume that too much information, especially about side effects, makes people anxious. In fact, the reverse seems to be the case. In surgery fuller information leads to fewer post-operative complications, with a quicker and less stressful recovery. In radiotherapy, it leads to greater knowledge about the treatment and less emotional distress (Audit Commission, 1993). A study of men undergoing elective surgery to repair an inguinal hernia found that a very detailed account of what might go wrong did not increase the patient's anxiety significantly and had the advantage of allowing patients to make a fully informed choice before they consented to surgery (Kerrigan et al., 1993).

If someone is about to undergo major surgery, it may help to talk to someone else who has faced a similar situation or been through a similar experience. Arrangements have been made by professionals in some hospital departments, where former patients talk to current patients before and after surgery. However, there may be conflicts between professionals and group members, as a study of a self-help group for patients after cardiac surgery found. When counsellors informed patients that they had felt depressed round about the third day after surgery and that this was common, some professionals disapproved. They felt this would become a self-fulfilling prophecy as there was no scientific reason for patients to become depressed. Members of the self-help group, for their part, resented the way some professionals dismissed their experiences (Simpson, 1996).

When making a decision, it is important to assess and compare the risks of each option, including the track record of the clinician and service. There are, for example, wide variations in the way different clinicians decide what treatment to give people with heart disease. One study found that 56 per cent of coronary artery bypass grafts were appropriate, 14 per cent inappropriate and 30 per cent equivocal. The proportion of appropriate bypasses varied from 37 to 78 per cent between different hospitals (Winslow et al., 1988). These differences may be important, but it can be difficult to find out about the competence of clinicians; this is maintained, in part, by the ethical code that does not allow doctors to advertise their skills or 'disparage' their colleagues.

Whether the decision is right or wrong in the end, what is most important is that it is the individual's decision. A study showed that emotional recovery after surgery for breast cancer was not related to whether the woman had had her whole breast removed (a mastectomy) or just the lump (a lumpectomy), but whether she and her partner felt they had made the decision. They may have followed the advice of the doctor, but it was their choice to follow the advice and to live with the consequences (Fallowfield et al., 1990). Other evidence shows that treatment is more successful, whether using physiological, behavioural or subjective measures, where patients participate more in the consultations with professionals (Kaplan et al., 1989).

People often do not feel that they are free to explore the different options for treatment or make a choice. Professionals may be assumed by patients to know more and to give impartial advice. By refusing their advice, it may appear that their professional expertise is not valued or that patients are not as ill or in as much pain as they say. If staff do not agree with the choices that individuals make, they may not offer them a choice (Lindow and Morris, 1995). Staff can undermine people's confidence by focusing on their impairments and not giving them the support they need to be independent. Furthermore, many consultations are rushed: the clinician is busy, with many more people to see. Even the most articulate patient or carer can find a consultation daunting and leave with questions unanswered. Some doctors are suspicious of articulate patients who turn up at a consultation with a list of questions. However, a study found that consultations were more efficient and effective when patients were encouraged to write down a list of questions they wanted to ask before the consultation. Patients raised more problems and the time spent on each of them was less (Middleton, 1995).

It is difficult to take in information in a short consultation, especially if it is bad news. Patients and carers may also be anxious, and may be given information in a way that increases their anxiety and affects their ability to

Information is needed to	User involvement	Getting users involved
Help people *use services better* • What services are available • How to use services	PASSIVE	• Consult users on content and style of information • Provide independent advocates (not just interpreters) • Ask users how services might be made more accessible
Improve health by providing *health education* on • Lifestyles • Specific conditions and diseases • Specific procedures and treatments		• Address problems defined by users • Offer solutions realistic in terms of people's lives • Provide counselling and support • Work with communities (see Chapter 5)
Enable *self-help* to assist people to live with and manage the condition better		• Provide independent funding for self-help groups to provide information and support to users
Make *choices and decisions* about treatment		• Provide independent clinical information, including outcome rates for units and consultants • Provide explicit standards so users know what they can expect • Offer interactive videos and CD-ROMs • Offer second opinions • Provide independent advocates (not just interpreters) • Involve users in setting and monitoring standards
	ACTIVE	

Figure 2.1 *Information for users*

understand what is said. A consultant surgeon in Brighton tape-recorded consultations with patients who had been told that they had cancer. They were encouraged to take the tape home and listen to it with someone else. It was found that 85 per cent of patients listened to the tape at home, almost always with someone else. More than a third said it contained information that they had forgotten (Hogbin and Fallowfield, 1989). Interactive videos and CD ROMs have been developed for some common conditions to give people information and help them make decisions. A pilot study of interactive videos on mild hypertension and prostate problems used in general practice found both patients and GPs reported favourably and that 71 per cent of patients reported the video helped them to make a decision about treatment (Shepperd et al., 1995).

It is important that people have as much information as they want – and understand it – so that they can decide for themselves, should they so wish. In developing joint assessment and care plans in mental health services, the Avon Mental Health Measure provides a good model. It was designed by users and professionals to help people assess how well they cope with many aspects of life – housing, money management, mood swings and sleep disturbance. This can be used to plan realistic and relevant care, and enables users to play a more active part in describing their own needs and the help they require (SW MIND, 1996).

Giving and receiving information can be seen as a continuum from patient education to individual autonomy. Figure 2.1 illustrates the different purposes that information may have and suggests how far users are involved or 'empowered' by it. Meredith (1993) carried out a study of patients' perspectives on participation and consent in surgery which showed that there had been changes in recent years: patients were asking more questions and professionals were responding to them. Nonetheless, he concluded that attempts to increase patient participation will continue to be frustrated:

> not simply because of a natural desire on the part of surgeons to reaffirm established professional rights to control the form and content of consultation, but because more demanding patients will disrupt the methods by which surgeons and other service providers have been able to fulfil the demands for patient throughput which a pressured health care system places on them. (ibid.: 315)

In other words, giving patients time to think over a decision could mean that more patients re-attend the clinic, thus taking up more time and putting more pressure on the service.

Some doctors look back with nostalgia to earlier times. This view is expressed thus by one doctor:

> I . . . urge caution in demanding more patients' choice in medical decision-taking. Will it make them happier, improve outcomes and fertilise, rather than sterilise, the delicate flower of the doctor–patient relationship? Unless it can be shown to be a widely applicable improvement by means of careful controlled trials of outcome, rather than simply recording patients' opinions, then I remain cautious about radical change. (Thompson, 1997: 4)

Controlling personal information

Health records are used to keep a record of diagnosis and treatment. They started out as a few personal notes, but are now seen as essential for audit purposes in order to provide consistent care to patients and to protect against possible litigation. Accurate and up-to-date records are also central to the working of the health care market; without them the purchaser cannot be accurately billed for tests and treatment, and providers will not be paid for the work they have carried out.

Medical records are assumed to be of universal benefit. However, there are difficulties from a user's perspective. First, records are not always a useful source of information. They may get lost and so treatment may be delayed while attempts are made to trace the notes. Notes themselves have become so detailed, with so many test results, that they are often too large and unwieldy to provide a coherent history or basis for a consultation. The hospital notes for an ordinary consultant outpatient clinic can be several feet high (Audit Commission, 1995).

Secondly, records hold personal and intimate information which people may not want to be widely known, and some of which may be embarrassing. Even though there are only a few circumstances where doctors have a duty to break confidentiality (normally when keeping it will put another person, such as a child, at risk), you can never be sure who will see the record or be told. Once information has been given to someone else, control of who else may be told will be lost and cannot be taken back. This can be important because, for example, a record of mental illness or alcohol misuse may mean you are not offered a job or have an offer withdrawn after the employer sees a medical report. A record of a test for HIV, whether it was positive or negative, may mean difficulty in obtaining insurance. Family members may not know about some health problems and you may not want them ever to know if, for example, you have had an abortion or a sexually transmitted disease. Even if these events happened long in the past and you change doctors, information remains on the medical record for the rest of your life. This deters some people from seeking help.

Thirdly, sometimes people feel that what is written in notes influences the way staff treat them. Once it has been suggested that you may have a mental health problem, drink too much or have marital difficulties, professionals may assume any symptoms, that cannot easily be explained, are to do with these problems rather than a physical cause.

Respect for confidentiality is a fundamental basis for trust between patient and clinician. Some people will only be willing to use services if confidentiality is guaranteed. People attending genito-urinary medicine clinics (clinics which treat sexually transmitted diseases) do not need a referral letter or to give their real name and no information is sent to their GP without their permission. This is because it is in the public interest to ensure that their infection is treated and they do not pass it on to other people. Similarly, women can seek contraceptive advice from a doctor who is not their normal 'family doctor' in order to preserve their anonymity.

Sometimes patients want to see what is written in their health records, which (except in private health services) belong to the Secretary of State. The Access to Health Records Act 1990 gave patients the right to see records about themselves that were made after 1991. However, access can be refused or information suppressed in certain circumstances. These include when it is felt that the information may 'cause serious physical or mental harm to any person' or 'would disclose information about an identifiable third party without his consent' (NHSME, 1990). Applicants may not know if information has been suppressed, even if they ask directly. The Act has its limitations, but has led to better record keeping and an increasing acceptance that records should be more open to the people to whom they refer. A survey by the Consumers' Association (1997a) found that though most people had little difficulty in obtaining access to their files, of those that did, one in four felt that they were incomplete or contained mistakes.

Patient-held records have been introduced in some services, such as for children and antenatal care, and could be useful for other people. For example, for travellers and people who move around, it is only patient-held records that are likely to be available when needed. Similarly, for people with mental health problems or chronic conditions who receive care from different health services and local authority social services, a patient-held record makes sure that everyone involved in the individual's care is kept up-to-date with what is happening, and it enables people to be involved and have more control over their own care. Patient-held records are also likely to be available in an emergency. For example, people with sickle cell disorders may have a crisis, go to the nearest accident and emergency department in excruciating pain and ask for painkillers. If staff do not know them, they may be suspicious that they are drug users and treatment may be delayed. If the patient can show a card, they may receive treatment more quickly.

Patient-held records can protect people's confidentiality. For example, people who are HIV positive may be reluctant to tell their GP about their status if they feel their HIV status will be put on their records and open for all staff in the practice to see. If the patient holds the record, they can decide for themselves who to tell about their HIV status. The GP can write on that record and so information on their HIV status does not need to be written on the health records kept in the surgery.

There needs to be a balance between respect for an individual's privacy and the need for full records in case of subsequent litigation or for child protection. In most circumstances the individual should be the 'owner' of personal information about themselves, and decide what information is disclosed – and to whom. There are arguments for and against patient-held records (Gilhooly and McGhee, 1991). These are outlined in Figure 2.2.

Disadvantages	Advantages
Patients lose their records.	Patients are less likely to lose records than hospitals.
Doctors may need to spend more time explaining the notes.	Patients benefit from better explanations.
Two copies of records may be needed, increasing the time and costs of producing and updating both.	Two copies are not always needed, although summaries and essential information should be held by provider.
Doctors may feel restricted and may keep another set of private notes.	A study found that clinicians were more likely to 'censor' diagnoses such as obesity rather than cancer or terminal illness.
Detailed information makes people more anxious.	Patients who are better informed tend to take more responsibility for their health.
Detailed information could destroy the rapport and trust between doctor and patient.	Studies show that patient-held records increase the rapport between GP and patient.
Records kept at home may be seen by other people without the permission of the patient.	Patients control the confidentiality of their records.
	Patients can correct any inaccuracies in their records.
	GPs can have access to notes on house visits, including records of hospital treatment.
	Records can cover both health and social care and improve co-ordination between services.
	Delays are avoided when patients move or change GP or attend an A and E department.
	Patients can keep their records longer than the provider may choose to.
	There are potential savings in storage and retrieval.

Figure 2.2 *Patient-held records*
Source: Hogg (1994) *Beyond the Patient's Charter: Working with Users*. London: Health Rights (adapted).

Missing patients – access and equity

A core value of the UK and European, but not the US, health care systems is that services should be available to everyone, regardless of their ability to pay or where they live. In spite of this, there are serious inequalities in access to health care and major barriers to using services – even with national systems such as the NHS. Some groups have greater needs for health care than others. Poverty, poor housing, and poor working and environmental conditions are closely related to ill health: death rates for people under 65 are four times higher in the poorest electoral wards than in the more affluent electoral wards. Children of unskilled parents are almost twice as likely to die in their first year than children of professional parents. There are great differences between the health of people from minority communities and those from majority communities. People from Pakistani and Bangladeshi communities are 50 per cent more likely to suffer ill health than whites. Much of the difference may be due to poverty as much as to ethnicity, since there are also wide differences between and within ethnic groups (Nazroo, 1997).

Potential patients, who might benefit, are missing out on health care. People from more disadvantaged communities are least likely to receive the type of health care they need. This is 'the law of inverse care' – those who need health care most are least likely to get it (Tudor Hart, 1971). In general, people who do not use services are those people who are unlikely to protest or express their anger.

Why people go 'missing'

There are many reasons why people miss out on health care. First, there are difficulties in planning and distributing services and skills equally in all areas. In some poorer areas and in inner cities there are fewer GPs or they are based in premises that cannot provide adequate facilities or services (Benzeval and Judge, 1996). Some people have problems in getting to and using health services, because of where they live or because they do not have access to transport or childcare. Specialist services are also disproportionately used by residents of the area surrounding the specialist centre. Sometimes these differences are important. For example, the alternative to treatment for end-stage renal failure is death. However, Dalziel and Garrett (1987) showed that the further people lived from a dialysis centre, the less likely they were to receive life saving treatment.

Secondly, some people seem to receive a poor service because of their age, race, disability, gender, class or lifestyle. This may be because of implicit and deep-seated attitudes that reflect the value put on people: that old people are less important than younger people; or that women are less important than men. For example, women are less likely than men to be offered cardiac surgery for the same condition (Petticrew et al., 1993). Older people also are often not offered services, including cardiac surgery and breast cancer screening (Pycock et al., 1995; Age Concern, 1996). Older people are more than twice as likely as those under 65 to die of heart disease and more than five times as likely to have a heart attack. Yet 20 per cent of coronary care units operate an age-related admission policy and 40 per cent of rehabilitation units impose age limits with no scientific basis (Age Concern, 1997).

Similarly with mental illness, patterns in diagnosis and treatment reflect how professionals see their clients. Black men in the UK are more likely to be perceived as dangerous by mental health professionals and far more likely to be labelled psychotic than white men. Black users of mental health services are three times more likely to be diagnosed as having schizophrenia than other users and less than half as likely to be given counselling – 32 per cent compared to 75 per cent of white users (Wilson and Francis, 1997).

Other people do not use services because of the prejudice they meet, or believe they will meet, if they do. HIV infection is connected in most people's minds with homosexuality, drug use and Africa. There is still an underlying distinction for many people between 'innocent' and 'guilty' people living with HIV. Haemophiliacs and babies are 'innocent'; gays, and drugs users and the people they sleep with are 'guilty' and so deserve what they get. Drug users with children may fear that if they ask for help with their drug problem or with financial or housing problems, social services will consider them unsuitable parents and take their children into care. Pregnant drug users may not go for antenatal care because of the attitudes of staff they meet, though antenatal care and managing drug use during pregnancy are essential to their health and that of their babies (Hogg et al., 1997).

A third reason why some people do not use services is because they are not what people want. There is a reluctance among many people to become involved with psychiatric services because they do not offer the sort of help they want. Some problems for people from black and ethnic minorities may be due to more than racism within services. Suman Fernando (1995) points out the great differences in perceptions of mental health between Eastern and Western philosophies.

Finally, some people do not know how to use services, what their rights are, or have difficulty communicating their needs and putting forward their views. There may be many different reasons for this: they lack information, English is not their first language, they use sign language or they are too ill to speak for themselves effectively. It is easiest to communicate with people most like ourselves. As many doctors are still white, middle class and male, women, poorer people, black and disabled people may have particular difficulties in communicating their problems to them. Problems in communication may cause distress to patients and their families but also may lead to inappropriate treatment.

Refugees and asylum seekers face particular difficulties in receiving basic services. They may have serious mental and physical health problems, some having survived torture, war, the stresses of flight from their own country, loss of family and friends, and adaptation to a new and very different country. Once they arrive in a country they are faced with housing and income problems. With little access to welfare benefits, their health and that of their children is likely to suffer due to poor food and inadequate housing. If you are homeless it is difficult enough to get access to health care; being a refugee or an asylum seeker causes additional problems and difficulties. Poor living conditions, homelessness and general ill health result in infectious diseases, such as TB, becoming a growing risk (Refugee Council, 1997).

Improving access

Improving access to health services requires changes in the way services are planned and provided to ensure that they are appropriate and acceptable to the people who will most benefit from them. The children of immigrants are able often to bridge different cultures and languages but are underused as professionals in health services. Medical appointments, in particular, have been shown to be biased and prejudiced. Esmail and Everington (1997) found this when they submitted identical applications for senior house officer posts from British trained doctors, half with Asian names and half with British names. The applicants with Asian names were less likely to be short-listed than those with British names. Refugees and asylum seekers have great health needs, and within these communities there are people with the skills and qualifications to provide services for them.

Wherever possible, ways should be found to enable people who have limited movement, speech, communication or intellectual abilities to speak for themselves. Advocates can help people who have difficulties in speaking for themselves to obtain information and put forward their views. The Association of Community Health Councils (CHCs) (ACHCEW, 1996) has argued that access to an independent advocacy service should be a right for all patients. The Mental Health Task Force set up by the NHS Executive included advocacy in guidelines on local mental health charters (NHSE, 1994).

While there is support for the principle of independent advocacy, there are no clear guidelines on who should provide advocacy or how it should work in practice. Many professions, especially GPs and nurses, have seen themselves as advocates for patients and see advocacy as good practice for all staff. After all, acting in the best interests of patients is an ethical responsibility for doctors and nurses. However, there is an important difference between advocates who are independent and advocates who are employed by the service. When advocates are not independent of the service, there can be a conflict of interest between representing both the client and the employer (McIver, 1993a). This presents increasing difficulties for voluntary agencies which have traditionally been advocates for users but now are themselves large-scale providers.

There are four forms of independent advocacy: legal advocacy, professional advocacy, unpaid lay or citizen advocacy, and self advocacy. Legal advocates have legal training and assist people to exercise or defend their rights through a local law centre or representation project, for example in a psychiatric hospital. Professional advocates speak on behalf of users and help people put forward their views. Citizen or lay advocates are generally unpaid volunteers who represent the individual's interests, independent of family, carers or health professionals. Volunteers are trained to work on a one-to-one basis in long-term relationships with people who may have learning difficulties or mental health problems. Peer advocates are people who have themselves used the service and who advocate for others using it. Self advocacy is where individuals are given support to present their own case and is used most by people with learning difficulties or mental health problems.

Advocacy schemes can help individuals get a better service and also improve services for others. For example, patients using bilingual advocacy schemes are more likely to feel that they can ask any questions about their medical care and to feel that the doctor has explained what will happen next (MORI, 1994). The City and Hackney Multi-Ethnic Women's Health Project was established in 1979 by the Community Health Council to help pregnant women, whose first language was not English, to understand the purpose of procedures in antenatal clinics and during labour and delivery, and to make their own decisions. With the introduction of advocates, non-English speaking women underwent fewer medical interventions (GLACHC, 1994).

Advocacy is an important right but relying on advocates has its dangers. Peter Beresford and Suzy Croft (1993) point out that the presence of an advocate may make other staff feel that they do not have to argue for the person's rights or develop the skills needed to enable people to speak for themselves. Professional advocates may feel that they have to present their clients in a negative light in order to make a stronger case for them in arguing, for example, for community care or disability benefits. Furthermore, advocacy may mean that people who are not represented are disadvantaged, thus confirming the low value placed upon them. Studies showed that, regardless of their case, people were more likely to win appeal tribunals if they were represented (Genn and Genn, 1989). Self advocacy also has its critics. The idea of self advocacy started with professionals and is itself a part of professional jargon. Self advocacy should be a part of all interactions, whereas the term may imply that trying to gain more control over your life is something that happens only at special times and in special places (Dowson, 1990).

There are enormous variations in access to and use of services – for many different reasons. When health services are forced to reduce growth in spending in the face of rising demand, 'rationing' services on the basis of individual characteristics could become an attractive option for some people. But this is a dangerous route where subjective moral judgements of the relative 'worth' of people rather than their clinical need may determine who receives treatment. People who do not smoke or are not overweight could be given priority – for example, for heart surgery. Services for people who are seen to create their own problems, such as drug and alcohol users, have always had difficulties in obtaining funding and may be particularly vulnerable. This lack of financial resources may also be justified in terms of effectiveness, since the evidence is that detoxification for drug and alcohol users often fails.

Every study of the use made of health services indicates that many people who might benefit are not receiving services. Missing patients enable savings to be made. Making services more accessible will increase demand so, rather than tackling these inequalities, it may be tempting to maintain them as a method of rationing. However, ignoring inequalities or allowing them to increase is short sighted. Evidence-based medicine should look not only at the effectiveness of individual treatments but also at who will most benefit. Missing patients need to be identified and services provided for them that they will be able to use.

Protecting patients and regulation

Patients are, by definition, vulnerable. They are worried about their health or are ill when they enter a strange environment where they may have little knowledge or expertise. Regulation is needed because patients do not have the same information as professionals who have incentives for over (and sometimes under) treatment. Regulation is also needed to ensure that services are provided to people who need them (not only to people chosen by the doctor) and are provided where people need them (not just in areas where doctors want to live and work).

Self-regulation

Traditionally the professions have been relied on to regulate themselves through bodies such as the General Medical Council and UK Central Council for Nursing, Midwifery and Health Visiting. Licensing was first introduced in England in 1512 when surgeons and physicians had to be licensed by the bishop or university in order to practise. The General Medical Council (GMC) was given official status in the Medical Act 1858. It holds the register of doctors, sets codes of conduct, deals with problem doctors and has the power to stop a doctor from practising. Though the GMC is set up by and depends on Parliament for its powers, it is funded by the doctors themselves which means that it is largely autonomous and free from external interference. In 1979 there were seven lay members on the GMC (out of a total of 93); by 1993 this number had increased to 11 and by 1996 to 25 (out of 104 members).

Self-regulation and professional freedom are based on the assumption that being a doctor requires an unusual degree of skill and knowledge, and so non-professionals are not equipped to evaluate or regulate them (Rosenthal, 1995). Professionals are responsible and may be trusted to work without supervision and, where necessary, to take action against colleagues. Out of respect for the principle of self-regulation, clinical judgement was excluded from the terms of reference of the Health Service Ombudsman when he was first appointed in 1973. Attitudes have now changed and, since 1996, clinical matters can be investigated by the ombudsman.

Professional self-regulation has serious inherent difficulties. Loyalty to the profession and colleagues is a central professional value, and doctors are restricted in how they can advertise their skills and services to patients. Until recently, the GMC regarded as 'capable of amounting to serious professional misconduct . . . the deprecation by a doctor of the professional skill, knowledge, qualifications or services of another doctor or doctors' (GMC, 1983). This was modified in 1989. Though the 'disparagement' of colleagues may still raise a question of serious misconduct, doctors have a duty to inform an appropriate body about a colleague whose behaviour raises a question of serious misconduct or whose fitness to practise might be impaired by a physical or mental condition (GMC, 1995).

In the 1980s the GMC was attacked from the right by enthusiasts for the health care market. David Green (1985), of the right wing Institute of Economic Affairs, argued that the health care market required that professional monopolies and restrictive practices be abolished. He suggested that the GMC should be replaced with a lay controlling body, concerned with market control rather than clinical standards. Green saw restrictive practices, such as the ban on advertising, as a way the profession maintained its status and income by stamping out competition. The ban on advertising was introduced in 1902 after a Dr Irvine accepted an appointment with a local charity in Birmingham. The charity put out a leaflet offering to treat the poor without charge. Dr Irvine was accused of infamous conduct for attracting patients away from other doctors and was forced to resign (Green, 1989). Not only do the restrictions on advertising keep competition between doctors to a minimum, they also give the profession an appearance of moral superiority over commerce. These restrictions also avoid the need to accept that users can make intelligent choices and have the right to do so.

In the 1980s the GMC also came under attack from patients' representatives led by Jean Robinson, a lay member of the GMC. She drew attention to the inadequacy of self-regulation in protecting patients from incompetent doctors (Robinson, 1988). Complaints from the public to the GMC were dismissed unless the complainant had substantial proof, so only complaints following a police or health authority investigation proceeded even to the first stage. Furthermore, the GMC only investigated 'serious' professional misconduct and so only covered the most flagrant negligence or behaviour. Professor Margaret Stacey (1992), who was also a lay member of the GMC, has described the reluctance of the GMC to look at clinical incompetence, which was not considered as important as other types of offences. Incompetence is not professional misconduct. While the number of doctors, complaints and court settlements have all increased, the number of cases taken on by the GMC has remained around the same. Marilynn Rosenthal sums the situation up:

> The rate at which cases are taken up is closely related to the resources available for their processing: staff, time, money, protocols. The GMC's review must always be constrained by resource limitations. Therefore, its functions are symbolic, signalling to both the profession and the public that it is the guardian of appropriate professional behaviour. (1992: 39)

By the 1990s the GMC sensed that the public had lost confidence in the way it operated. It sought powers, under the Medical (Professional Performance) Act 1995, to take action against doctors where there is concern about their competence and the standard of their practice, without the need to identify a specific incident of serious professional misconduct. The GMC increased the proportionate number of lay members and included the appointment of lay people to teams which assess a doctor's performance under the new performance procedures. It is also setting clinical standards and protocols within which doctors will be expected to operate (Irvine, 1997).

A turning point may have been reached in 1998 when the General Medical Council found three clinicians guilty of serious professional misconduct following the deaths of 29 babies at the Bristol Royal Infirmary. It appeared that, for a number of years, children undergoing heart surgery there were more likely to die than those having operations in other regional units, because of skills failures and a lack of expertise among these surgeons. Staff in the hospital who were concerned were either unable to do anything or were ignored (Davidson, 1998). Eventually an anaesthetist blew the whistle and, belatedly, action was taken following a television programme. The anaesthetist was forced out of his post and went to work in Australia in order to continue his career.

Hospital doctors have their own procedures and so are rarely subjected to GMC disciplinary procedures. These hospital-based disciplinary procedures have been used in professional disputes, unrelated to patients' concerns. In 1986 Wendy Savage, a consultant obstetrician and gynaecologist, was suspended from clinical practice following the death of a baby. The reason was that she had a different approach to maternity care than her (male) colleagues. She provided services in GP surgeries and encouraged women to have a say in how their babies were delivered. At the inquiry it was shown that the perinatal mortality rate for babies in her care was lower than that of the professor who had accused her and was responsible for bringing the inquiry. She was completely exonerated. In *The Wound and the Doctor*, Glin Bennet (1987: 66) summarized this: 'It is a classic case of individual conduct being so threatening to the tribe that the person concerned must be eliminated by any means, yet the precise nature of the crime cannot be stated explicitly. Therefore some charge has to be found: virtually any charge will do.'

Where professionals dominate, as in the UK, the main interest of the regulatory bodies is professional misconduct rather than clinical conduct and there is a reluctance to impose severe sanctions. The GMC revokes considerably fewer licences than either the American or Swedish boards (Rosenthal, 1992); interestingly, in Sweden and the USA, regulation and licensing are undertaken by public bodies not by the profession. In Sweden the licensing board has a majority of consumers and maintaining clinical quality (rather than behavioural propriety) has been the major concern. This is perhaps a more effective approach to raising standards and protecting patients than concentrating on professional misconduct. The question is how to identify and assess inappropriate practice early enough to protect patients. There are many different problems that can lead to mishaps – such as alcohol or drug use, mental health problems, inability to work with colleagues, ignoring the views of patients or plain incompetence. Effective arrangements to protect patients need to recognize these different problems and develop effective ways of dealing with them.

An important feature of effective regulation is a culture that emphasizes that managers and professionals owe a moral duty to users and not only to the organization or their profession. Staff face serious problems in seeking to report situations where they feel that patients are being abused. In the 1990s there was a culture hostile to whistle-blowing at all levels. The management style, stress of work and short-term contracts meant that people felt unable to express their views without risking their jobs and careers. People were asked to leave, often with only time to clear their desk, and had clauses in their severance contracts requiring their silence (Bruggen, 1997). In 1997 the Labour Government announced legislation to protect whistle-blowers: the Public Interest Disclosure Act 1998. This, with a Freedom of Information Act, could lead to a shift in NHS culture.

In the long term, a clinical audit that relies on systems of peer review and co-operation in order to raise standards is likely to be the most effective way of protecting patients. Nevertheless, external controls are needed to ensure that peer review does not degenerate into reaffirmation of professional solidarity.

External regulation

With increasing doubts about professional self-regulation, other ways of protecting patients developed: internal inquiries after mishaps, service specifications by purchasers, public scrutiny through community health councils, complaints procedures, and clinical audit, disciplinary procedures and external auditors such as the Audit Commission. External regulation generally involves an element of policing and is normally developed in reaction to particular events. The NHS Health Advisory Service (then the Hospital Advisory Service) was set up by Richard Crossman in 1968 as a direct result of revelations about staff cruelty in long-stay hospitals. It was set up to improve the management and standards of care for mentally handicapped, mentally ill and elderly patients in England and Wales, and to advise the Secretary of State about the conditions in hospitals. Community Health Councils (CHCs) were set up as public watchdogs on local services in 1974. The Audit Commission was set up in 1983 to audit local health services and is concerned with 'value for money'. The Social Services Inspectorate was set up in 1985, as part of the Department of Health, in order to promote best practice for implementing government policy and to report to the central department on local developments. The National Audit Office looks at the functioning of government departments. These bodies are expert bodies providing a mixture of professional consultancy, inspection and setting standards, with little user or public involvement. There are other regulatory mechanisms, such as the Medicines Control Agency and the Embryology and Human Infertility Authority, that have close links with the industry or are largely funded by the industries they regulate. Users are not normally involved.

In 1998 the Labour Government proposed a new system of clinical governance that would ensure that clinical standards were met, with NHS trusts having for the first time a statutory duty for quality. It proposed a Commission for Health Improvement to support and oversee the quality of clinical services and tackle shortcomings, with powers to intervene directly when a problem is identified but is not being tackled. Members of the Commission are to include patient representatives. In addition, a National Institute for Clinical Excellence was proposed to draw up new guidelines, emphasizing clinical and cost-effectiveness (Department of Health, 1998a).

External regulation is particularly important where professionals have a direct financial interest in the transaction with the patient. Though the need for regulation is greatest in private services, the present legal framework for registration and inspection of private facilities is complex and unwieldy, with some statutes going back to the National Assistance Act 1948. Registration and inspection of hospitals and nursing homes is carried out by health authorities and local authorities under the 1984 Registered Homes Act. Prospective providers are required to prove that the carers working in the home are fit to do so and that the premises are suitable. Given limited resources, the present system of public inspection is often more an administrative process than effective control. The result is that only the worst abuses are likely to be discovered. A survey found that one in ten carers of people with Alzheimer's disease said that their relatives had been mistreated in residential or nursing homes. The mis-treatment included restraint, rough handling, neglect of personal hygiene, poor standards of feeding and lack of stimulation (Alzheimer's Disease Society, 1997).

There is little evidence to suggest that either self-regulation or external regulation are effective by themselves as a deterrent to incompetent practice. Power (1994) has argued that audits do not automatically mean that organizations are more open to scrutiny. People may attempt to manipulate the system to meet the standards or to satisfy auditors. The existence of the audit makes people subject to audit act in such a way that the case for external audit is made even stronger. For example, monitoring waiting lists may lead to ways of keeping the number of patients on waiting lists down, without actually treating more patients. The response to the failures of audit has been to demand better and more detailed scrutiny and audit, rather than to look at the reasons for the failure.

Dissatisfied patients – complaints and redress

If you are dissatisfied with a product or service you have two options: you can stop using the service and go elsewhere; alternatively you can complain or express your views, in order to try to get the service you want or obtain redress. In health services most people neither have the option to go elsewhere for the service, nor find it easy to voice dissatisfaction. Complaining patients do not fit into the medical model of the doctor–patient relationship and staff often have an emotional resistance to accepting the right of people to complain, in particular in 'free' public services. People are not expected to complain about gifts they receive. Making a complaint, however, is a central consumer right and fits into the consumer model.

NHS complaints procedures to 1996

Complaints from users have been the basis for much regulation, but would-be complainants face many problems. Patients are generally ill and vulnerable, entering an alien and complex system run according to rules that they may not know or understand. In addition, they may not know what standards they should expect or how to complain; they may feel that complaining will do no good and may get them into trouble. Not surprisingly, many complaints are made on behalf of other people: children, elderly parents and even neighbours. There are particular problems for mental health service users because of the psychoanalytic tradition that discounts and explains away clients' views as symptoms of their illness. As a result patients who complain may be dismissed as manipulative or displaying signs of their illness. If their carers complain, this too can be dismissed as guilt or a part of the family dynamics which have contributed to the illness.

When the NHS was set up, it had been intended to establish a system for inspection and complaints, but this did not happen because of opposition from the medical profession (Webster, 1996). The need for a complaints procedure surfaced again in 1969 when a report on the abuse of mentally handicapped patients in Ely Hospital was published and caused a scandal. Following this the Davies Committee published a report on hospital complaints in 1974. The report recommended a national code of practice for dealing with suggestions and complaints about hospitals. However, hospital and community services were not required to have a complaints procedure until the Hospital Complaints Procedure Act 1985 was passed, but this Act did not specify any particular standards. A national complaints procedure for hospitals, community services and family practitioners was finally introduced in 1996.

Until 1996 the would-be complainant was faced with a complex array of procedures. The procedures were based on different models: the prosecutory/disciplinary model and the consumer-oriented/learning model (Allsop and Mulcahy, 1996). The complaints procedure for family practitioners (GPs, dentists, pharmacists and opticians) was based on a prosecutory/disciplinary model, where the aim was to establish fault and blame and not to satisfy the complainant's grievance. It was set up as disciplinary procedure by Lloyd George's Government in 1911 to investigate breaches of contract, which were mainly disputes brought by insurance companies about charges and sick notes. Complainants were expected to pursue their complaint through a formal adversarial procedure and produce evidence and witnesses, even though they did not have equal access to medical records or witnesses.

There were separate procedures for hospital and community services. These were, at least in theory, based on a consumer-oriented/learning model where the purpose was to satisfy the complainant and for the organization to learn. However, in general, staff were often concerned with appeasing the complainant rather than investigating the complaint or seeing how services might be improved. Complainants had no right to see information and there were no standards for the investigation of the complaint. If local procedures failed, complainants with grievances about clinical care in hospitals could ask for an independent professional review of their complaint by two consultants from other hospitals. However, it was up to the hospital manager to decide whether a complaint was to be referred for independent professional review and the regional health authority to decide whether to arrange a review.

In fact the way that complaints were handled sometimes made complainants more dissatisfied, rather than resolving their grievance (Department of Health, 1994). The National Association of Health Authorities and Trusts (1993: 9) summed up the problems: 'The arrangements are seen as over-complex, failing to be user-friendly, taking too long, often over defensive and often failing to give any satisfactory explanation of the conclusion reached'.

The problems with the procedures became increasingly apparent as complaints increased. The number of complaints more than doubled in

England between 1982 and 1991: from 16 218 to 32 996. But in the year following the launch of the Patient's Charter in 1991, they increased by over 25 per cent (to 44 680) (Department of Health, 1994). This perhaps reflected the publicity around the Charter and the replacement of the ethos of the compliant patient with that of the consumer.

The new NHS complaints procedure

Because of these concerns, the government initiated a review of NHS complaints procedures. The subsequent report by the Wilson Committee identified principles for complaints procedures and the features of an effective procedure (Department of Health, 1994). The principles were: responsiveness to complainants, using complaints to improve services, cost-effectiveness, accessibility, impartiality, simplicity, speed, confidentiality and accountability. The principles were in line with those on which voluntary organizations and consumer groups had campaigned and were, in general, supported by them.

Following this, in April 1996 a new complaints procedure for all NHS services was introduced. Under the new procedures staff aim to deal with the problems and difficulties of patients as they arise ('local resolution'). If local resolution fails, complainants can ask for an independent review of their complaint, where a panel with an independent chair and clinical assessors investigates the complaint. If complainants have been refused an independent review or are dissatisfied with the outcome of the review, they may ask the Health Service Commissioner (ombudsman) to investigate their complaint. The jurisdiction of the Health Service Commissioner (which previously excluded complaints about clinical matters and against family practitioners) was extended to include all NHS complaints.

Turning the principles of the Wilson Report into reality has proved difficult. There were a lot of problems in the first year following the introduction, some of which were due to the haste with which it was implemented. A survey by the Consumers' Association (1997b) found that the system was not operating as it was supposed to. Six out of ten respondents were not satisfied with the overall handling of their complaint, its final outcome or how long it took to resolve.

The challenge, the National Consumer Council (NCC, 1993: 7) noted, was to turn the NHS into 'the kind of organisation that welcomes complaints at every level and can persuade its consumers that "it's OK to complain"'. The success of the procedure depended on the attitudes and training that staff received, but investment in training was limited. However, the new procedures did act as a catalyst for change. One hospital found that some complaints could be prevented if the senior nurse on a ward asked each patient on each shift how they were and dealt with problems they had at an early stage (Beecher and Coochey, 1997). Correspondence following this report in the *Health Service Journal* pointed out that ward sisters used to see talking to patients as part of their job.

Other problems emerged that were inherent in the design of the new system (NCC, 1997). Many people do not want to talk to the staff involved about their complaint and this deters them from complaining. If the complaint is about sexual abuse or serious negligence, talking to the staff concerned is quite inappropriate. As a result the more serious complaints may not come to light or be investigated. There were particular problems within general practice, where there was no monitoring of how practices handled complaints. People who made a complaint could also find that they, and other family members, had been removed from the practice list; making a complaint was seen by the practice as evidence that the doctor–patient relationship had irretrievably broken down.

It also proved very difficult for people to obtain an independent review. Only one in eight requests for independent review were granted in the first year (Buckley, 1997). Additionally, the procedures have turned out to be bureaucratic and costly, which may mean they come to be seen as 'not cost-effective' or unaffordable. Effective complaints procedures are an important consumer right and an essential part of ensuring consumer participation and satisfaction in the health service. They provide important information for improving services and may avoid the major costs of litigation. However, the costs of investigating complaints are easier to identify than the benefits for an individual or an organization of a good complaints system.

Some user groups are concerned that complainants have no part in the new disciplinary procedures for family practitioners, which they did have before. If disciplinary action is taken, the investigation of the complaint finishes. This means that complainants may not obtain the explanation they wanted or find out what happened. Complainants may be called as witnesses, but they have no right to information or to know the outcome of disciplinary investigations. If they are not called as witnesses they may not even know that a disciplinary investigation is under way. This is in contrast to their rights in General Medical Council (GMC) hearings which are held in public and where the complainant has legal representation, normally paid for by the GMC. Knowing what action is taken is very important for some people. They may be left with the feeling that justice has not been done or that what went wrong has not been adequately explained.

Many people are in private nursing or residential homes paid for by the NHS, but are not covered by NHS complaints procedures. In private hospitals and nursing homes, many patients are isolated and vulnerable and it is difficult for them to complain about staff who will continue to care for them. The Mental Health Act Commission (1995) expressed concerns about the way complaints in private care were handled. It reported that the investigation of complaints in private nursing homes was generally undertaken by the hospital manager, who rarely found in favour of patients. The Commission recommended that private nursing homes should review their procedures in line with the Wilson Report and that, for serious incidents, they should bring in an independent investigator – as occurs in special hospitals (Mental Health Act Commission, 1995).

Legal redress

Redress comes too late. The patient has already suffered and services have failed. Litigation is the main way of seeking redress in health care for both publicly and privately funded services. In deciding whether there are grounds for legal action after a mishap, people need information about what has happened. However, people are not supposed to use the complaints procedure to get the information they need to decide if there are grounds for litigation. If it is thought that a complainant may have a case for litigation, staff may be even more reluctant to be open – in case they give information that could be used in subsequent legal action. The Wilson Committee pointed out that poor handling of complaints may mean that people feel that they are forced to resort to solicitors to get the answers they want.

Legal action is stressful, costly and time-consuming for claimants. If successful, they may not receive a settlement for many years after the accident. However, when a person is disabled or looking after someone with a disability, they need money immediately. Michael Bolger was a victim of medical negligence which resulted in him becoming a paraplegic and being confined to a wheelchair at the age of 47. He wrote:

> Pursuing litigation can generate a wide range of negative emotions, including feeling undervalued and cheapened because few people appear to place any importance on what has happened to you; overwhelmed and alienated by the legal procedures and terminology used and by the legalistic stance of the defendants; vulnerable and insecure because of the risk of failing; and isolated because of the absence of an independent support network. (Bolger, 1996: 6)

When after five and a half years his case came to court, the health authority admitted unconditional liability within two weeks of the start of the hearing. He was awarded £1 675 000. He had spent a total of £310 000 pursuing the claim.

Litigation has only been an option for those with a significant disposable income or who have legal aid. Solicitors may, however, now take on cases of personal injury caused by medical accidents on a conditional fee ('no win, no fee') basis. Conditional fees were introduced for personal injury and medical negligence claims in 1995 and medical negligence may be excluded from legal aid in future. Conditional fees may work where the cause of injury and person responsible is clear from the start, such as in a road traffic accident. But in medical negligence the causes and the people responsible are often very difficult to establish and the success rate is low. It may cost £6000 or more to obtain expert reports and other services, simply to find out if you have a case at all.

Furthermore, claimants would need to be protected from paying the legal costs of the other side should they lose. This is normally done by 'after-the event' insurance policies – and the premiums can be very high for medical negligence. As a result, relying on conditional fees may give better access to justice for a few but will remove the possibility of litigation from many people (Bawdon, 1997).

All hospital negligence awards since 1995 have been met out of the NHS budget and, when judgement is delivered, hospitals have to pay the compensation immediately. John Harris (1997), a professor of medicine, law and ethics, has suggested that it is inequitable to give successful litigants absolute priority in the sharing out of NHS resources. Victims of medical negligence who win large compensation awards against the NHS should take their place in the queue for scarce resources, he suggests. Successful litigants should have their needs assessed and go on a waiting list for payment only when there are no more urgent claims to be met. This could lead to a situation where a successful litigant might never become a priority and, therefore, never receive the compensation he or she had been awarded.

There are particular problems in obtaining redress for damage caused by drugs. No cases against drug companies have come to court, though there have been out-of-court settlements for drugs such as Opren and Thalidomide. To succeed in a claim against a drug manufacturer, you must prove that the drug was defective and that this caused the injury. However, even if you can prove these, the company can put forward a defence that it is not reasonable to expect the specific defect to have been identified, given the state of knowledge at the time. This defence based on 'development risk' was introduced in the Consumer Protection Act 1987. Had it been available at the time of the Thalidomide case, the pharmaceutical company might have used this defence to argue that it could not be expected to discover that the drug gave rise to foetal malformation early in pregnancy. It might even have won (NCC, 1991).

The rising costs of litigation and compensation claims, and the difficulties faced by victims of medical accidents, led to interest in the no-fault compensation schemes which operate in New Zealand, Sweden and Finland. Under these schemes claimants are required to prove that the injury was the result of an accident or mishap, but not that it was due to negligence. The case is reported to a central body which investigates and awards compensation where appropriate. Though some schemes have run into financial difficulties and problems in determining who is eligible, no-fault schemes provide a speedy and simple way of getting compensation. Though compensation awards tend to be lower, more people receive compensation.

However, critics have pointed out that such schemes make it difficult for people to find out what happened to cause the mishap and do not hold professionals to account (ACHCEW and AVMA, 1992). Often people take legal action in order to establish the truth and find out who was to blame.

They are not simply looking for compensation. The difficulties with no-fault schemes can be seen in the case of children with cerebral palsy, who make up around eighty per cent of successful litigants. Lamb and Percival (1992) point out that, since it is difficult to prove the cause of cerebral palsy, a no-fault scheme would not necessarily benefit children with cerebral palsy. Most cerebral palsy is caused either during pregnancy or after delivery in very immature babies. In general, only fifteen per cent or so of parents of children with cerebral palsy could sue because the damage occurred during or around the birth; eighty-five per cent of parents of children with cerebral palsy could not.

There is increasing use of mediation to avoid litigation. Successful mediation may meet complainants' desire for information and recognition, while avoiding high legal costs. An alternative system for providing compensation is a comprehensive disability income scheme that provides support on the basis of the fact of injury or disabling condition, without needing to find out how it was caused. This is supported by disability organizations and is considered to be fairer since the level of compensation is determined by need not by the cause of the mishap. However, it would be important to ensure that incompetent or negligent practitioners were still called to account.

Buying health care

In the 1980s and 1990s there was a growth in private health care. Concerns about waiting lists, and overworked and overstretched services have encouraged people (and their employers) to take out private insurance and opt for private health care. Following the organizational changes in the 1990s, many patients in private services are publicly funded through referrals from health authorities and GPs.

Before the NHS, doctors obtained their income from private patients, who subsidized the public work they did in voluntary hospitals. Dr Julian Tudor Hart described it thus:

> Doctors traditionally recognized two kinds of patient. Paying patients, like other customers, were always right and therefore had to be humoured. Non-paying, public service patients, were supposed to earn their right to care by having serious or at least interesting diseases, and to be grateful for getting any care at all; beggars can't be choosers. (1994)

Patients who pay can choose which practitioner they see and, to some extent at least, set terms for the consultation. If they are not satisfied they can refuse to pay or can find another practitioner. Patients in public services often feel that they can only exercise choice in a passive and negative way – by 'non-compliance' and by ignoring instructions. Those with money can make more positive choices.

Some people choose complementary therapies, including homeopathy, osteopathy, herbal medicine, acupuncture, chiropractic and massage, as well as self-care approaches such as meditation, yoga and relaxation. There has been a rapid rise of these therapies recently. In the past, the deep-seated antagonism of the medical profession to non-conventional treatments polarized orthodox and unorthodox clinical practice. Only fifteen years ago many considered them to be for cranks. Up to the 1980s the British Medical Association's (BMA) handbook of ethics stated that doctors should not refer patients to osteopaths. As a result, people may use complementary therapies but do not tell their doctor: they do not want to face their disapproval.

However, the distinctions between orthodox and complementary therapies are being broken down as a result of the market and consumer pressure. It is estimated that one in four of the population has used some form of complementary therapy (Stone, 1996). About sixty per cent of health authorities and forty-five per cent of GPs either commission or provide complementary therapies, though the total amount is very small in terms of overall NHS spending (Adams, 1995; Thomas et al., 1995). The growth of alternative therapies has been mainly in the private sector, and so most are not available to people on low incomes, including many with chronic conditions and disabilities.

Some people seek alternative therapies because conventional medicine has failed to solve their problems. However, Rosalind Coward (1989) argues that the popularity of alternative approaches reflects wider changes in attitudes. If the reason people go to alternative therapists is because they find orthodox health services mechanistic, bureaucratic and un-caring, the people using alternative therapies would surely have tried to change orthodox services. But, on the whole, the pressures to make orthodox health services more user-centred have come from the rise of the health market and consumerism.

There is no question that many people want complementary therapies and find them helpful. Conventional medicine often has little to offer people with long-term or intractable problems, and they like the more gentle and holistic approach of alternative therapies which gives them a sense of worth and well-being. However, the further integration of complementary therapies with conventional approaches is inhibited by two factors. First, there is little systematic research on the benefits of complementary therapies, and research does not normally use self-esteem and well-being as criteria in assessing the outcome of treatment, except for psychological treatments. Assessments of clinical and cost-effectiveness need to take account of the importance of self-esteem in helping people cope with their ill health or disability and also the savings that may be made in the drugs bill.

Secondly, there is little regulation of practitioners or arrangements for protecting people who use complementary therapists. The consumer magazine *Health Which?* has recommended that therapists' professional bodies should set minimum standards, have a code of practice, and complaints and disciplinary procedures as well as insisting that members have professional indemnity insurance (Consumers' Association, 1997c).

Anyone can buy medicines and health products over-the-counter in a pharmacist, supermarket or health food shop. The range of drugs, previously only available on prescription, is increasing – in line with several other European countries where many drugs, including antibiotics and oral contraceptives, are available over-the-counter. Self diagnostic kits are also readily available to test for pregnancy, cholesterol and blood pressure levels; and the range of tests is increasing, including genetic testing. In this way people can bypass the doctor, and diagnose and prescribe some remedies for themselves. The market for over-the-counter medicines is potentially vast. Over any two-week period, nine out of ten adults will report having experienced at least one ailment. Non-prescription medicines are used to treat one in four of these episodes (Blenkinsopp and Bradley, 1996).

Being able to diagnose problems, choose medicines and bypass professionals gives people more control and enables them to take more responsibility for their own health. But they need independent information to be able to do this, which is not always so easy to find. Traditionally it has been up to the provider to produce information for patients, now commercial companies are providing information to patients about conditions and procedures. Drug companies are targeting the public through advertising on TV, information leaflets, helplines, links with user groups, and the Internet; they are even setting up 'support' groups to provide information to patients. A Consumers' Association survey (1996) found that leaflets for patients about medicines failed to mention important side effects and did not help people understand how drugs work or manage their condition.

Poor quality information involves risks since some over-the-counter medicines may be dangerous, even if taken correctly, if the patient is taking a prescribed drug at the same time. The Consumers' Association (1996) found that six in ten people with asthma and half of those with high blood pressure had taken non-prescription medicines that they should have been warned to avoid. For example, painkillers that contain aspirin or ibuprofen can trigger symptoms in people with asthma. Pharmacists can advise customers; however, they are in an ambiguous position as they are professionals but also business people who make their living from selling medicines.

Health Action International, a consumer group based in Amsterdam, wants to see tighter controls on advertising. A study by the International Organisation of Consumer Unions found that most advertisements to the public did not meet the ethical criteria laid down by the World Health Organization (IOCU, 1994a). Most did not mention any side effects in the marketing copy, which added to the impression that over-the-counter drugs are safe. There is a danger that expensively produced glossy literature is little more than covert advertising for a particular product or associated treatment regime (Meredith et al., 1995).

Self medication is seen as a way of shifting some of the cost of drugs to consumers. Though obtaining medicines over-the-counter may save some consultation time for doctors, it may not reduce costs for the NHS because so many people are exempt from prescription charges and will still obtain them through their GP (Thomas and Noyce, 1996). The greater availability of drugs over-the-counter may lead to an increase in the over-all consumption of medicines, which is comparatively low in England and Wales. In 1989 in France the average person received 38 prescriptions, in Italy 20, and in Germany 12; in contrast, in Britain the average number of prescriptions was 7.6 and in the Netherlands it was 6.9 (Audit Commission, 1994). This difference may be due to the incentives for prescribing given to doctors in insurance-based health schemes, compared to publicly funded health services in the UK and the Netherlands. The Audit Commission noted that there is no conclusive evidence that higher drug expenditure leads to better health. In fact, increased drug consumption has dangers.

The demand from consumers has led to a growth in private health care, both in orthodox and unorthodox medicine. This has advantages for users in increasing the diversity and choice available to them and encouraging them to take more responsibility for their own health. Patients or consumers who pay have a superficial advantage but face the same problems as other patients. There are very strong commercial reasons for controlling the information available to consumers, and manipulating them to use their consumer power to buy particular services and particular products. This means that regulation is increasingly important as part of consumer protection (Gilbert and Chetley, 1996).

There are also dangers in the increased reliance on private health care, both for the individual and for public health. First, it may lead to increased drug consumption, inappropriate treatment and even harm, because of the commercial incentives to offer treatments to those who can pay irrespective of clinical need. For example, the Office of Fair Trading in 1996 noted that private patients could be having unnecessary operations, including heart surgery and joint replacements.

Secondly, stimulating demand can lead to inequalities in access to health services. Choice may become accepted as being about the add-on extras for those who can afford to purchase them but which are not available to people in the publicly funded system. Choice may be between a private room with a telephone and a mixed sex ward. However, it can also mean the difference between a competent and experienced surgeon and a trainee; or between a rundown psychiatric unit that relies on mind altering drugs and a supportive therapeutic community or long-term psychotherapy. Commercial providers are also concerned about meeting the wants and not the needs of patients. As Pfeffer and Coote (1991: 24) put it: 'Commercial enterprises seldom need to worry who exactly their customers are, or whom they should satisfy, as long as people can afford to buy in sufficient numbers, at the right price, to assure profitability'.

Campaigning patients

Campaigning for patients' rights began in the USA in the 1960s and 1970s when it was recognized that consumers needed rights, information to exercise their choice, and protection in the market economy. Patients' rights movements paralleled the women's movement, the civil rights movement in the US and the self-help movements which emphasized the importance of speaking for oneself and valued people's own experience over professional knowledge. In the UK, the consumer movement developed with the establishment of the Consumers' Association in 1957 and the government-funded National Consumer Council in 1975. Many voluntary organizations were set up in the 1950s, 1960s and 1970s questioning established professional practice, often with support from radical professionals. Community health councils (CHCs) were established as part of the NHS in 1974 to represent the views of local people to managers.

Campaigning thrives on rhetoric and a colourful language that pushes for radical and idealistic changes that can only be achieved, if at all, after a struggle. Charters are a good way for groups to express their values and aspirations. In the 1980s the first campaigning patients' charters were produced in the UK. These included the Charter for Children in Hospital produced by NAWCH (the National Association for the Welfare of Children in Hospital) and now Action for Sick Children in 1984; the Patients' Charter produced by the Association of Community Health Councils for England and Wales in 1986.

Since then many voluntary organizations have produced their own charters, which reflect the issues of most importance to them. Some of these reflect basic human rights, where people feel that by using health services they will experience discrimination and their rights as citizens will be jeopardized, in particular people with mental illness, learning difficulties or who are living with HIV. Others, such as charters for people in chronic pain, emphasize the importance of staff attitudes and respect for the patient's autonomy. Charters have also been important in campaigning internationally. The UN Convention on the Rights of the Child, which was ratified by the UK government in 1991, and the European Declaration on the Rights of Patients of 1994 are both important milestones in developing an international framework for rights (see Chapter 7).

In 1991 the government took over the concept of charters. The Patient's Charter, which was published in England in 1991, was a mixture of unenforceable rights and undefined standards. It encouraged people to expect certain standards from health services in the same way as they would in other services. The Charter was about promoting information and choice and linking the ideology of the individual consumer with the organizational changes of the market. Furthermore, there was widespread public concern about the proposed health service 'reforms' and the Patient's Charter was seen as a way to reassure the public that they would benefit from changes.

There are problems in applying the concept of rights to health care. Most charters are a mixture of rights and standards. A 'right' is any claim or title that is morally just or legally granted as allowable or due to a person. Rights should be enforceable by law, while standards are aspirations which will not always be reached (Plant, 1989). In practice, definitions may not matter since rights in health care are largely symbolic and few are enforceable in law. For example, an individual does not have the *right* to health care. While the Secretary of State has a duty to provide a comprehensive health service, this right is not enforceable in law. In 1987 the parents of Baby Barber went to court to try to secure an injunction on a hospital to perform a heart operation on their child for which the hospital lacked funds. The court took the view that the limitation of funding was a matter for politics rather than the law (Hughes, 1991). The right for one person to have treatment, say a kidney or heart transplant, may mean that someone else is denied that right. After all, there are only a limited number of skilled staff to carry out the surgery and a limited number of organs available for transplantation.

Some rights are hard to define and depend on who is defining them. For example, definitions of the right to privacy and to be treated with dignity will depend on who is making them, their expectations and experiences, and will be different for people from different cultures and communities. The right to give informed consent raises problems in practice in defining what is 'adequate' information. The law is more often used by professionals to override the right to informed consent than by individuals asserting their rights.

In general, voluntary organizations and pressure groups were suspicious when their campaigning language was taken over by government in the Patient's Charter. The first concern was that the Charter was published with little consultation and did not necessarily reflect the areas that users felt were most important (Hogg, 1994). However, once standards were in the Charter, priority and resources were given to them – often with unexpected results. For example, the number of people waiting for treatment and the length of time they wait are, at first glance, important and easy to measure. The Patient's Charter gave people the right to be admitted to hospital for virtually any treatment within two years of joining the waiting list. As a result people were treated on the basis of the length of time they had waited rather than on their clinical need. By giving all conditions equal priority, waiting times may be shortened for less important conditions but lengthened for conditions where delays matter.

The second concern of patients' organizations was the lack of independent monitoring of the implementation of the Charter. The implementation of some parts of the Charter was monitored and the information published as 'league tables'. Almost inevitably this may mean that those standards included in league tables may be given more resources than other areas – some of which may well be more important to patients. For example, improvements in the time people wait to see a doctor in outpatient departments may lead to shorter consultation times, with less time for explanation and information. League tables for the number of complaints may not actually show how satisfied or dissatisfied patients are, but how willing the service is to accept and record complaints. League tables may provide a disincentive to services to have an open and positive approach to complaints.

Following the launch of the national Patient's Charter, local services, including GP practices, were required to produce their own charters. Though initially charters may be a catalyst to change, they are not necessary to improve standards. Standards need to be explicit and negotiated with staff and users as part of an overall quality programme, but this does not require a charter. Furthermore, the language of rights and responsibilities does not fit well in the individual relationship of patient and professional. It is aggressive and implies conflict, and so may introduce a tension that neither patients nor professionals want. Not surprisingly, there was a backlash which resulted in the replacement of the Patient's Charter with a charter for the NHS, giving patients responsibilities along with their rights. The emphasis has changed from 'empowerment' to 'partnership' which is less threatening and antagonistic to professionals (NHSE, 1996b).

Moving on to look at ways of giving consumers real power, John Spiers, at one time a NHS trust chair and later Chair of the Patients' Association, has argued that patients must be given control over money: 'If we genuinely do want empowerment and consumer choice, there is no alternative but for patients to be given the compelling power of money. This will wrest substantial control over financial mechanisms away from managers as well as physicians' (Spiers, 1997: 64). This could be done by giving patients vouchers to choose where and how they receive health care. A voucher is not normally a piece of paper, but an accounting category which defines the amount of money that is transferred to a provider for a particular service used by the entitled individual. Saltman and Otter (1995) outline two types of vouchers. There are vouchers which are a general entitlement to a nominal sum to purchase a particular service (such as dental care or maternity services). Alternatively the voucher can be differentiated according to the recipient's income or need and calculated individually or by category. Capitation fees in general practice may be seen as a form of payment by voucher, since the GP receives a set payment for each patient, with an increased amount for older patients who may take up more time.

The use of vouchers in health care is limited. Vouchers may work where there is a fixed need which can be quantified and budgeted, such as housing or childcare, and where the service is physical in nature and can be inspected, monitored and evaluated. In health care a fixed price on the value of the service the individual receives tends to restrict the range of services available and creates incentives for providers to select less costly patients or to reduce the quality of the service. Because of the incentives to under-serve voucher holders, there would be a need for strong regulatory and monitoring mechanisms. Some of these difficulties have been seen in general practice, where there are reports that a few general practices refuse to register patients – or even remove them from their lists – if they require costly drugs, make demands on staff time or make a complaint. Saltman and Otter concluded that vouchers disempower patients; it is difficult for individual patients to hold providers, who are paid by vouchers, accountable for their decisions – particularly privately capitalized providers. The provider also loses public accountability as the public funder does not have management authority over the provider. Finally, the costs of the administration and regulation of voucher schemes need to be considered.

Conclusions

Doctors may be partly magicians, relying on their craft and status, and partly technicians, relying on their skills and science to help patients. Patients may be partly compliant, wanting responsibility taken from them, and partly consumer, wanting to choose the product and its quality – and reserving the right to complain if they are not satisfied. Individuals may find themselves acting sometimes as a compliant patient and sometimes as an irresponsible one, both perhaps within a single consultation. People may follow advice and take the medicines prescribed for a heart condition, but continue to have an occasional cigarette or cream bun. Compliant patients may become dissatisfied and complaining patients, sometimes because they put their trust in professional expertise and feel betrayed when the results are not what they expected. In most patient–professional consultations there may be aspects of consumerism alongside the paternalism of the past. Tension would appear to be inevitable where the clinician and patient enter a consultation with different assumptions about the consultation and what they can expect from each other.

  The relationship of doctors and patients has changed in recent years. Health care is often no longer the intimate relationship of the doctor and patient of the paternalistic model, but involves health professionals working in multi-disciplinary teams as well as with family carers. As the traditional authority of the medical profession is undermined and patients become more confident, a different basis for the contract between the giver and receiver of health care is needed. Ultimately the relationship of health professional and patient needs to be based on mutual trust

	Paternalism	*Consumerism*	*Partnership*	*Autonomy*
Values	Principles of good medical care override individual treatment preferences and values. Concern for patient overrides efficiency.	The patient's health care values dominate. Efficiency and effectiveness are considerations.	Values of professional and patient are negotiated and agreed. It is recognized that some patients are disadvantaged in access to services. Efficiency and effectiveness are considerations.	The different perspectives of patient and professional are recognized, but the patient's health care values dominate. It is recognized that some patients are disadvantaged in access to services. Patients and carers may demand treatments against the evidence.
Goals	Doctor and patient have common goals to promote patient's health. Doctor retains power and has high status.	Doctor and patient have divergent goals: • the patient wants good health as he or she defines it • the doctor wants appropriate treatment for the patient, as he or she defines it, in addition to money and status.	Doctor and patient have common goals based on joint assessment agreed during the consultation.	Doctor and patient have common goals negotiated during the consultation, but patient's preferences prevail.
Relationships	Doctor has obligations and patient has needs.	The patient has rights: the relationship is equal or patient may have greater power.	The patient has rights and responsibilities.	The patient has rights and responsibilities.

	Paternalism	Consumerism	Partnership	Autonomy
Relationships (continued)	Enduring relationship between patient and doctor. The patient does not complain.	The patient shops around for services, while doctors market their services.	The inequality between patient and professional is recognized as well as the need for advocacy.	The inequality between patient and professional is recognized as well as the need for advocacy.
		The patient will complain or seek redress if dissatisfied.	Patients can complain, but this may lead to a breakdown of the partnership.	Patients can complain and this is accepted as a right.
Decision making	Doctor has more expertise and power and makes the decisions.	The doctor gives information and the patient makes the decision.	The doctor gives information and the decision is made by the patient jointly with the doctor.	The doctor gives information and the decision is made by the patient. The doctor respects the patient's right *not* to follow professional advice.
Accountability	Self-regulation is a professional matter.	Legal accountability for medical errors, which may lead to more defensive medicine.	Clinical standards are audited and reviewed according to national standards.	Clinical standards are audited and reviewed according to national standards.
	Patient does not hold doctor responsible for bad outcomes and mistakes.	External regulation and policing may be required as consumer protection.	Regulation involves professional and lay people.	Procedures for independent investigation and regulation to protect patients.
	Third party intervention is inappropriate.			Redress available for victims of medical accidents.

Figure 2.3 *The doctor–patient relationship – different models*

between equals, and involves professionals and patients redefining what they mean by 'best interest'. Different models proposed to replace paternalism are summarized in Figure 2.3. Each of these models, however, raises problems.

Consumerism sees the individual as a consumer in the marketplace. The consumer looks for the best deal and may not feel loyalty to a particular 'brand'. The motto is 'let the buyer beware'. Being a consumer also requires having choice. However, having choice depends on whether the professional is willing to offer choice and whether the NHS is prepared to pay for it. People may feel powerless in relation to health services compared to other services because they may be anxious and vulnerable when seeking or receiving health care and do not want to be seen as 'difficult'. Consumerism does not take account of the complexity or intimacy of the professional–patient relationship and the importance of trust in that relationship. The 'myth' of patient as consumer is discussed further in Chapter 8.

Partnership recognizes that people should be encouraged to be as involved and take as much responsibility for their treatment and care as they want (Williamson, 1992). Both parties have knowledge and must co-operate to provide effective health care: patients are not necessarily autonomous or dominant. However, 'partnerships' require equality and sharing of the benefits and the risks, which is not the case in health care (see Chapter 8 about the 'myth' of the patient as partner).

Autonomy sees the individual as an equal with the clinician, free to decide his or her own goals and to act according to those goals. Professionals respect each individual even if they disagree with their views or actions. 'Autonomy' shares some of the problems of consumerism; it may not deliver equity and may even increase inequalities. People who are in a position to negotiate for themselves may benefit, but more disadvantaged people will not. 'Autonomy' may also lead to ineffective treatment, since what the patient and his or her carers want may not be based in evidence of effectiveness or priorities for public health.

These models do not explain the way people behave when they are seeking or receiving health care. Professor Patrick Pietroni (1996) suggests that the individual's beliefs, needs and expectations determine how people seek health care. First of all there are the basic survivors – patients who are barely surviving, overburdened by family, financial and housing problems. Their demands may be couched in physical terms but their needs are often psychological, economic, social and spiritual. They form a dependent relationship with the GP and want pastoral care. Then there are the conspicuous consumers who want convenience, choice and for the service to operate as an efficient supermarket. They seek information so they can get the best buy and are often influenced by fashion and the latest medical advances, such as annual cholesterol tests. Finally, there are the self-actualizers who want explanations and information. They wish to be more involved in their health care and accept more easily a psychological and spiritual explanation for their disease. Their focus is towards empowerment and fulfilment, and, increasingly they want to be involved in the ethical and moral debates surrounding medical procedures. These three types, Pietroni suggests, fit into Maslow's theory of the hierarchy of needs. Only when their basic needs are met, are people able to become consumers or self-actualizers.

It is important to go beyond the rights of the individual to look at social rights and issues of equity, otherwise many people from disadvantaged communities may continue to be excluded. Empowerment and sharing power are widely used words, but often with little understanding of the complexity of the processes involved. People who have power are not always aware of their power and may not use it, but those who do not have power are well aware that they do not have it. Achieving a more equal relationship will require patients and carers to have more information available to them as well as the confidence to use their knowledge. The sort of services that might result from a user-centred health service are outlined in Part III.

3

HEALTHY PEOPLE

Health is an episode between two illnesses.

Dr Ted Kaptchuk (1986)

Health is a state of complete physical, mental and social well-being, and not merely the absence of diseases or infirmity.

World Health Organization (WHO), Constitution (1948)

Many things affect our health – where we live, where we work, how we live, the food we eat, the air we breathe, our genetic inheritance, the germs we come into contact with. Most of us are going to live with disease and disability for large sections of our lives, and so awareness of our health and what we should do to keep healthy preoccupies us more and more. In the nineteenth century social reformers and sanitarians successfully reduced deaths by improving housing and working conditions and by providing clean water. The medical profession were not initially involved but soon took public health over, away from the engineers and the city planners. As a result public health moved from changing the environment in which people lived to approaches that relied on clinical interventions, such as screening for disease and immunization programmes, or attempted to change the way people behaved through health education. As medicine was seen to be more effective in curing disease, it began to have more importance and people looked to clinicians to solve many more of their problems. Preventing diseases by controlling the social circumstances and environments that caused them became less important. Medicine, taking this view, could compensate for an unhealthy environment or lifestyle.

In this chapter health promotion, screening and immunization – and the ethical issues they involve – are considered.

Promoting health

Much of the time we take our health for granted. We live our lives, taking risks with our health – whether by overworking, overeating, or taking drugs or alcohol. Some of us may see ourselves as healthy when we have no identifiable disease or symptoms, or as long as we are able to function adequately. Alternatively we may see ourselves as healthy when we feel fit in mind and body and so feel able to cope with what life throws at us. Seen from this viewpoint, health is like a reserve of capital – one which can be diminished by self-neglect and increased by healthy behaviour (Blaxter, 1990). Health education programmes encourage us to take better care of ourselves in order to increase this 'health capital'. More and more our feeling of well-being is determined by how much we do to promote our own health. A research project into people's attitudes towards their health found that none of the people interviewed were suffering from any 'treatable' illness, yet almost all described themselves as 'not really healthy' on the grounds that they did not do enough for their health (Crawford, 1985).

Women and children have been the main targets of health educators and of screening and immunization programmes. Women are more likely to worry about their own and their family's health than men, perhaps because of their role in the family. However, men's health is becoming a popular topic in the media, including calls for 'equity' in screening for male as well as female cancers.

Health education

Health education began with the public health movement in the nineteenth century, with emphasis on the importance of cleanliness and hygiene in controlling infectious diseases. However, now the messages tell people how to avoid risks to their health and attempt to stop them doing things that they may enjoy – such as smoking, unsafe sex, drinking alcohol or using drugs. Health education has traditionally been seen as a question of professionals passing on information to the public and expecting them to comply in the same way they are expected to comply in individual consultations. There are several reasons why this approach has not been very successful.

First, health education messages are complex and often based on con-flicting sets of evidence, which may undermine them. For diseases such as cancers, heart disease and strokes, no simple causes have been identified and so there are no simple messages for health education campaigns. For example, campaigns for preventing heart disease are based on 'risk' factors such as smoking, diet and lack of exercise. But 'risk factors' do not predict who will develop heart disease: heart attacks can come with no warning to those without risk factors. Older people remember how fre-quently health education messages change. In the 1930s 'healthy' foods included butter and sugar. These then became 'unhealthy' and were replaced with 'healthy' substitutes; now people are told these may have their own risks. They were told that alcohol was bad for them, but now are told that red wine may prevent heart disease (though it may contribute to breast cancer).

Secondly, health education tends to concentrate on the 'risks' that the individual takes and ignores the risks imposed on them by society. Health education to prevent breast cancer has focused on risk factors such as diet, while the risks involved in taking oestrogen in the contraceptive pill or hormone replacement therapy or arising from exposure to pesticides, for example, are ignored. For heart disease, factors such as stress, race and social class may be more important than smoking, diet or lack of exercise (Farrant and Russell, 1986).

Thirdly, health education campaigns sometimes fail because they do not take into account why people act as they do. Young people take risks; changing what they do now out of fear of getting cancer or heart disease in twenty years time hardly seems a priority to them. Also there are reasons why individuals drink too much, take drugs, eat unhealthy diets and smoke; they do not do these things in isolation. For example, pregnant women are a major target of anti-smoking campaigns. Ann Oakley (1989) concluded that pregnant women continued to smoke in full knowledge of effects on the baby as a way of coping with their difficult circumstances. She also questioned why health educators target smoking and not diet in pregnancy, both of which affect the birthweight of the baby. She concluded that diet depends more on the woman's income and so is outside her control. Women may have different priorities. Judgemental attitudes of health educators may make their decisions more, rather than less difficult.

There have been changes in approaches to health education, in particular in the need to combat HIV infection and substance misuse. Media advertising about drugs, by itself, is not only ineffective but may even encourage young people to experiment with illegal drugs by inadvertently glamorizing them (Advisory Council on the Misuse of Drugs, 1984). People will take risks, whatever information they are given, and they need to be encouraged to reduce these risks. So campaigns promote safer sex not abstinence, and provide drug users with free syringes and needles so that they do not have to share needles and thus risk being infected with HIV. This pragmatic approach makes some people uneasy as they feel it condones illegal or immoral behaviour.

The Health of the Nation (Department of Health, 1992) launched a strategy in 1992 in England to cut preventable diseases, with 27 targets for the NHS to reduce coronary heart disease, stroke, cancer, mental illness, HIV/AIDS and accidents. Health authorities were given responsibility for meeting the targets. Though health professionals can improve the uptake of screening programmes and run health education campaigns, they have limited influence on health education in schools. Similarly, health professionals cannot make changes to improve the environment; government policies on poverty and low income, poor housing, unemployment and the environment are more important in promoting public health. The government can also influence behaviour by drink driving laws and restrictions on drinking. Price rises (through tax increases) and restrictions on smoking in public areas are likely to be more effective than health education or counselling.

Many of the targets in *The Health of the Nation* were not met. People are getting fatter and more younger people are smoking. It was recognized that it was necessary to widen the basis for the national public health strategy. In 1998 the Labour Government published *Our Healthier Nation*, a Green Paper that reviewed the strategy laid out in *The Health of the Nation* and put it in a wider context of inequalities in health (Department of Health, 1998b). This approach acknowledged the effect of structures and the environment on lifestyles and looked beyond health and illness in the narrowest sense (such as morbidity and mortality rates) to developing 'healthy living centres' addressing issues such as welfare rights, housing, community safety, inequalities and even 'well-being' – sketching an ideal vision of how people might live. There was disappointment, however, that targets remained attached to reducing deaths from specific diseases rather than reducing inequalities.

Health education failed in the past because the messages and the methods were selected by professionals, without consultation with the people they sought to influence. Some health promoters now recognize that working with communities is more likely to be effective in encouraging people to avoid risks and change their habits (Chapter 5).

Health promoting products

Sometimes it is difficult to distinguish health promotion campaigns from the advertising of health products. As healthy eating and diet are seen as more and more important, an enormous health food and diet industry has developed. The lines between over-the-counter medicines, vitamins, nutritional supplements and food are becoming more and more confused. The 'discovery' of a so-called ideal weight means that many people are identified as overweight and as having a health problem. Foods may promise to make us thin and also may promise us health. There is also a growing food industry that uses health promotion to market its products. Some foods may be marketed for people with particular conditions, such as sugar-free foods for diabetics or gluten-free products for people who are gluten intolerant. Other products are promising to slow the effects of ageing or to enhance physical or mental performance; for example, in Japan a fortified soft drink has been targeted at adolescents facing school examinations. The market for health promoting products is based on creating a demand for commercial products among people who might otherwise feel they are healthy and excludes those who cannot afford to purchase these benefits.

Screening

Screening is another growth area. In 1995 private screening services increased by 24 per cent (Laing's Review of Private Health Care, 1997). Medical centres in high street shops and railway stations offer cancer screening and cholesterol tests. Screening for disease identifies people who have specific conditions. It has two functions: early detection to prevent the spread of disease and protect public health; and early diagnosis of diseases or conditions. Early diagnosis of disease or particular conditions may be expanded to discuss some specific issues pertinent to antenatal screening and genetic testing.

Protecting the public

The origins of screening lie in the state's interest in protecting healthy citizens. Screening for disease was initially used as a 'sieve' to separate healthy and useful people from the unhealthy and useless ones (Skrabanek and McCormick, 1989). For example, lepers were segregated for centuries and quarantine was imposed on prospective immigrants to the USA. Some screening for insurance companies or employers still serves to filter out the unhealthy from the healthy; the person who is likely to make a claim on the insurance company from those who are less likely to.

Doctors are legally required to notify the Department of Health when they have a patient with a particular infectious disease, such as typhoid, meningitis, measles and food poisoning, based on legislation dating back to the nineteenth and early twentieth centuries. People who are carriers, though themselves unaffected, are prohibited from taking on occupations where they might infect others such as in catering. There was a famous case in the USA of a woman known as 'Typhoid Mary'. She was a carrier and worked as a cook in the houses of the rich. She left a trail of death and disease behind her in houses where she worked between 1900 and 1907. When the connection between the presence of Mary in the house and the disease was recognized, attempts were made to prevent her working in kitchens. However, these were not successful; she had to earn a living and cooking was the only way she knew how to do this. In the end she spent the final years of her life confined to a hospital to prevent her from infecting other people.

Calls for screening to protect the public from people with infectious diseases have also arisen in response to the spread of HIV infection. In 1987 the US Senate voted unanimously to mandate HIV tests for all applicants for legal immigration to the US; the governors of three states – Minnesota, Texas and Colorado – signed laws permitting local authorities to quarantine indefinitely HIV positive individuals who seemed to pose a threat to society because of their sexual activities. Belgium, West Germany, Greece, Finland and Spain all passed new legislation or interpreted pre-existing public health law to permit the expulsion of, or deny visas to, HIV positive foreigners who were seeking work permits or to study. These laws were primarily directed against Africans and, in Germany, against Turks. In February 1987 a US Army sergeant was sentenced to four years in prison by German authorities for knowingly spreading the disease to his sexual partners (Garrett, 1994). In November 1987 the President of the German Federal Court of Justice announced that, in the absence of an HIV vaccine, it might soon prove necessary to tattoo and quarantine people who were infected with the virus. The last time that Germany had carried out tattoo and quarantine measures on its citizens was during the Second World War when 'misfits', Jews and other undesirables were placed in concentration camps.

Coercion made no difference to the spread of the virus. Apart from the implications for citizens' rights, such laws are difficult to enforce and only discourage people coming forward for testing or for treatment. Discrimination simply drives AIDS underground and thus encourages its spread.

Early diagnosis

Through screening, signs of disease can be picked up and treated earlier, sometimes preventing serious illness or death. The self-evident benefits of screening have become a part of our general belief system. In surveys of what people want from health services, health check-ups and screening come high on the list (Consumers' Association, 1987). However these 'wants' may not always be justified by any evidence that they provide benefits (Dowell et al., 1996).

Screening was initially introduced for diseases such as TB which had a known cause and an effective treatment. Now screening is offered for diseases where causes and treatment are less well understood: heart disease, specific cancers and prenatal defects. The screening programme for cervical cancer, for example, was introduced in England in 1964 and it seems to have had little impact on mortality rates from cervical cancer. In a study of nearly a quarter of a million women in Bristol, ranging over a twenty-year period, the death rate in 1992 was shown to be similar to that in 1975 when continuous screening was first introduced (Raffle et al., 1995). Generally the failure of screening programmes to deliver the expected benefits is blamed on poor organization and the poor technical quality of screening programmes. However, the central dilemma remains: it is not known how many women with a harmless condition are being treated with lasers or given hysterectomies. Cervical cancer, which is a relatively rare cancer, has become a major health concern for women, often causing unnecessary distress (Posner and Vessey, 1988).

In retrospect the cervical cancer screening programme may have been developed before there was evidence that it would be effective. In spite of this, few of the lessons of cervical cancer screening were applied to breast cancer screening, which was introduced in 1988. There are problems in the accuracy of the screening test for breast cancer. Wright and Mueller (1995) note that about five per cent of women who are screened for breast cancer have positive or suspicious results, but that most of them (80–93 per cent) are false positives. For women who are screened and no abnormality is detected, between ten and fifteen per cent actually have the disease. The number of women referred to services with false positive results causes delays in treatment for women with diagnosed breast cancer. As it is, around ninety per cent of breast cancers are discovered by women themselves and not through screening programmes (Austoker, 1994). Wright and Mueller (1995: 29), writing from a public health perspective, concluded: 'since the benefit achieved is marginal, the harm caused is substantial, and the costs incurred are enormous, we suggest that public funding for breast cancer screening in any age group is not justifiable'.

In spite of the uncertainties surrounding cancer screening, often health education literature on breast cancer and cervical cancer screening has been misleading. Information published does not include the risks and possible adverse consequences of screening or make it clear that it is not able to prevent the disease or guarantee a cure. Until 1995 there was no mention in leaflets about cervical cancer that there were any problems with the efficacy of the test.

For some people screening may mean that cancer is diagnosed earlier, but for others it causes unnecessary anxiety and even means they have unnecessary treatment. Screening and 'false positives' continually remind people of their mortality and can make apparently healthy people feel that they might be in the grip of a terrible killer disease – cancer – even though they feel well. There are calls for more resources and better monitoring of standards, but there is no discussion of abandoning mass cancer screening, which would be unpopular with the public and politically unacceptable. It is just hoped that new diagnostic techniques and better treatment will eventually mean that screening programmes can deliver the promised benefits. There are frequent calls in the media by professionals for more screening programmes, including for prostate cancer. This is despite evidence that there is uncertainty about the accuracy of tests for prostate cancer and despite a lack of certainty as to whether treatment actually prolongs life. The latter is particularly important because many men find that they are impotent and even incontinent after treatment (Adami et al., 1994).

Antenatal screening

Pregnant women generally find that screening by ultrasound and blood tests are acceptable and reassure them that their baby is healthy. Ultrasound is particularly popular as parents feel that seeing their baby helps them to bond. Tests can identify a foetus which may have an inherited disorder and then parents can choose to terminate the pregnancy if they want to. However, diagnostic tests, amniocentesis and chorionic villus sampling (CVS) can only rule out a few specific conditions. None guarantee that the child will be healthy, nor are the tests always accurate. For example, a study in Denmark found that there had been an increase in the number of foetuses diagnosed with Turner's syndrome (Gravhold et al., 1996). This is a disorder that results in short stature and failure to develop breasts and ovaries in girls. Three quarters of mothers who were given this diagnosis chose to terminate the pregnancy. The researchers found that 32 in 100 000 baby girls were born with the condition. However, after amniocentesis or CVS, it was being diagnosed in 176 foetuses per 100 000. Of the mothers who chose to continue with their pregnancy, 8 out of 13 babies tested after birth proved to be normal.

Antenatal tests do not comprehensively prove anything about a baby's health or prevent babies having a disability. If tests show that a foetus has a disability, a termination, often by inducing labour early, may be recommended but this is a solution many parents do not want. Furthermore, disabled people point out that this approach implies that they should not have been born. People with disabilities and their families may be stigmatized, if they choose to opt out of screening programmes. Joanna Moorhead concludes that the result of these trends is:

> the level of anxiety among pregnant women is rising, and what should be nine happy months looking forward to motherhood are being eaten away with worry waiting for test results and scan appointments. Some women, facing a termination if the test result shows an abnormality, refuse to allow themselves to acknowledge their pregnancy until the all-clear comes through, sometimes at well over half way through. (1996: 114)

Genetic testing

Screening is available for inherited single gene disorders – cystic fibrosis, thalassaemia and sickle cell disorders. Couples can find out if they are carriers of the gene and what the chances are that their children will be affected by these disorders. Kits for a genetic test for cystic fibrosis are already commercially available. You can send samples to be tested to find out if you have the gene and you will be sent the results, with an offer of counselling. Genetic testing may help some people to plan their future and decide whether to have children.

However, the knowledge that you will develop an incurable disease may be hard to live with. There is a test for Huntington's disease (also known as Huntington's chorea), an inherited degenerative disease of the nervous system which develops when people are in their thirties or forties. In Britain only a few hundred of the many thousands of people who know themselves to be at risk of carrying the Huntington's gene have come forward since the test was first offered in 1987. For some people, uncertainty is easier to live with than the certainty of a degenerative incurable disease (Jones, 1994). Similar issues are faced by people in deciding whether to have an HIV test, though their position is further complicated by the virus being an infectious disease which they can pass on to others.

Genetic screening for susceptibility to diseases such as the common cancers, cardiovascular disease and diabetes may soon be technically feasible. Genetic screening may be able to provide each person with a profile of their tendencies to develop particular diseases. In the USA there have already been attempts to market a test for the predisposition for breast cancer, but this is being resisted by professionals. However, even if you are susceptible, it does not mean that you will develop the disease or even indicate when the disease might develop. Knowing your susceptibilities may just cause distress to you and your family, and change the course of your life unnecessarily – especially given the inaccuracy of many clinical predictions. However, life and health insurance companies may demand that applicants are screened so that people with a high risk of particular diseases can be refused insurance or charged higher premiums. Someone could have a genetic test as a teenager and it may affect their whole life – partnerships, families and getting a mortgage (NCC, 1995). Genetic disease is one of the contingencies that people should not be expected to protect themselves against. One result of this may be that the principle of a publicly funded health service, where the risks are shared by all people equally, might become more politically acceptable again.

Focusing on genes also blames the 'victim' rather than looking for wider causes that may contribute to people being susceptible to particular diseases. It may distract attention away from environmental factors that contribute to disease. For example, there are genetic conditions which are related to occupational diseases; some employers in these fields may prefer to screen potential employees so that people susceptible to particular occupational diseases are not employed, since this might be cheaper than cleaning up the workplace. The causes of disease would then be blamed on the individual characteristics of workers rather than on the industrial environment. Social and political measures may be more appropriate than screening individuals and persuading them to modify their lifestyles.

Screening for genetic defects and susceptibility raises ethical dilemmas. Where will the testing of unborn babies stop? Testing for gender in India and China is already leading to the abortion of female foetuses and, consequently, serious imbalances in the ratio of males to females. This is having major effects on society as children reach puberty. In future it may be possible to test for intelligence or for a 'gay gene'. Genetics as a science is relatively new but its origins lie in eugenics, which was the practical application of Darwinian theories of evolution. Eugenics was founded by Francis Galton, Darwin's cousin, in order 'to check the birth rate of the Unfit and improve the race by furthering the productivity of the Fit by early marriages of the best stock'. Many eminent Edwardians supported the principles. In 1913 the Mental Deficiency Act introduced compulsory certification for people admitted to institutions as mentally defectives, and this was the basis for excluding them from other welfare and social agencies as well as from the general education system (Ryan with Thomas, 1997).

Sterilization of 'inferior' people was introduced throughout Scandinavia and in most states in the USA. In Germany during the Nazi regime there were programmes to exterminate people with mental and physical disabilities; later, people from particular ethnic groups, such as Jews and Gypsies, were targeted. German laws were tougher but they were in line with trends elsewhere. Though no sterilization law was introduced in the UK, there is some evidence that enthusiastic public health doctors encouraged voluntary sterilization of 'defective' people in their areas in the 1930s (Webster, 1997). Genetics may have moved beyond these dubious origins and have an enormous potential to give a better under-standing of disease and ill health. However, human genome research is being conducted in a commercial climate, and there are profits for those corporations that can develop and patent tests and techniques ahead of their competitors. This could lead us to go back to supporting the notion that genetic endowment is the main determinant of health rather than material circumstances such as poverty (Clarke, 1995). The lessons from the recent history of genetics need to be borne in mind when planning genetic screening programmes. People personally affected by genetic disorders need to have a voice in these debates.

Immunization

The spread of some infectious diseases can be prevented by immunization, which involves inoculating people with a substance derived from a particular bacterium or virus. This encourages the body to develop antibodies to the disease. The practice of inoculating people against small-pox, which caused one in twelve deaths in eighteenth-century London, is ancient. In the West of England there was a traditional belief that an attack of cow pox gave protection against smallpox. The first vaccination (after the Latin word for cow, *vacca*) was carried out by Edward Jenner in 1776 when he inoculated a boy with matter from cowpox vesicles and six weeks later with smallpox. The boy did not develop smallpox. Jenner published his discovery that vaccination with cow pox produced immunity from smallpox in 1798. Smallpox vaccinations were compulsory in the UK from 1853 until 1948.

Many immunization programmes rely for their success on universal coverage – 'herd protection'. The theory is that if enough people are immunized against a particular disease, it will eventually disappear, as has happened with smallpox worldwide. This benefits poorer families who are more likely to live in inadequate and overcrowded housing, where infectious diseases flourish. Children in poorer families are also less likely to be healthy or to receive prompt and good medical care when they are ill. The main immunization programmes for childhood illness were introduced relatively recently: diphtheria in 1940, polio in 1956, whooping cough in 1957, measles in 1968, rubella in 1970 and the MMR (measles, mumps and rubella) in 1988.

There is, however, a conflict between benefit for the individual and benefit for the community as a whole. Through immunizations healthy people, especially children, are put at risk of adverse reactions to the vaccine, when there is no way of knowing if they would have developed the disease or its complications. Occasionally children have neurological damage from immunizations used in child health programmes. When there is publicity about problems resulting from immunizations, parents may not have their children immunized and this can lead to outbreaks of the disease. Between 1977 and 1979 and between 1981 and 1983 there were rises in the number of cases of whooping cough when public anxiety meant that many children were not immunized.

There are pressures on parents to have their children immunized. In many countries, such as the USA, children must be immunized in order to enter school. In France, child benefit is dependent on the parent producing proof that the child has been immunized. In the UK the pressures come from incentives to doctors rather than to parents. GPs can receive additional payments of several thousand pounds if 90 per cent of the children on their list are immunized.

At what point does this persuasion become coercion? Publicity about adverse effects has made some parents, quite understandably, reluctant to immunize their children. These are difficult decisions for parents. Adults can choose to ignore advice and live with the consequences. However, when you are choosing for someone else, such as a child, the decision to ignore professional advice is harder. The information given to parents aims to reassure them about the safety of immunization. For example, rubella is usually a minor illness, except for in pregnant women when it can harm the foetus; there is no benefit for boys to be immunized at all, but this is not always included in information for parents. The assumption seems to be, possibly rightly, that if parents know the full story they may be less likely to have their children immunized.

Parents and professionals may calculate the risks of immunization quite differently. The risks in epidemiological terms may be minimal: but if your child is the one who has permanent brain damage, you would have preferred to take the risk of whooping cough. Dissent is getting stronger. Some parents have set up support groups to give other parents information and help them to resist the pressure to have their children immunized. Parents who want such information are finding it easier as they can have access to the same information as professionals from the Internet.

At the point where more information to the public means less compliance, it is time to reconsider the whole programme. There comes a point in all programmes where the risks of immunization outweigh the benefits. For example, smallpox was eradicated from the USA by 1950 and after that the risk of complications from the vaccination was greater than that of catching smallpox. In the 1960s, studies showed that each year following vaccination seven to eight people died and hundreds had complications, two hundred of whom had to be admitted to hospital (Russell, 1986).

Ethical issues

There are confusions and ethical dilemmas in providing health services to apparently healthy people. When people are ill, they seek help from clinicians. The relationship is clear: they need professional expertise and are generally grateful. When people are encouraged to put themselves in the position of patient, even though they have no obvious health problem, the relationship is different. Professionals are selling something to people which they have not asked for. In 1971, Archibald Cochrane and Walter Holland wrote:

> We believe there is an ethical difference between everyday medical practice and screening. If a patient asks a medical practitioner for help, the doctor does the best he can. He is not responsible for defects in medical knowledge. If, however, the practitioner initiates screening procedures he is in a very different situation. He should, in our view, have conclusive evidence that screening can alter the natural history of diseases in a significant proportion of those screened. (Quoted in Holland and Stewart, 1990: 18)

Preventive programmes should, therefore, offer clear benefits and enable people to make informed decisions. However, by participating in preventive programmes, people incur risks as well as benefits and programmes are not always based on uncontroversial evidence of benefit. The public are generally not encouraged to exercise their right to give their informed consent.

Screening, immunization programmes and health education induce a feeling that health is something that cannot just be accepted when we have it, but must be worked for. The more attention we pay to our body, the more we notice, the more symptoms we can spot and the more important they seem. We may even blame ourselves and feel guilty if we develop a disease, feeling that we might have prevented it if we had only tried harder. People are encouraged to worry about their health and even seek help from doctors when they feel well. If they can afford it, they may pay for services or products that may improve their health. This can lead to people becoming the 'worried well'. Targeting resources on healthy people also means that there is a danger that the people with the least health problems make totally disproportionate demands on health services, increasing the inequalities in access to health care between the rich and the poor.

At one end of the continuum are the 'worried well' who are unnecessarily concerned about their health. At the other are the irresponsible people who take no heed of advice and so may incur blame. Health education ensures that most people know the 'right' behaviour, but sometimes – in fact often – people carry on smoking, drinking alcohol and eating fattening foods. What responsibility does society and the health service have towards people who choose to put themselves at risk? Should an irresponsible person compete on equal terms for treatment with other people who do not indulge in risky behaviour or have looked after their health? Judging people on the grounds of their lifestyle may be dangerous, since health and susceptibility to disease are complex and little understood. Some people, though not many, find it easy to give up smoking or lose weight. For others it feels impossible and the costs are too high. The reasons for bad habits and unhealthy lifestyles go deeper than even the environment, income or stress levels. There may be a genetic susceptibility to addictive behaviour, such as smoking, under or overeating, drug and alcohol use. Genetic susceptibility may determine which smokers get lung cancer and which do not. The reasons for 'irresponsibility' run deep and touch on basic ethical issues.

Another ethical dilemma is the balance of benefit for the individual and to society as a whole. How far should individuals be persuaded or coerced to comply with public health programmes, such as the fluoridation of water supplies, screening and immunization programmes? There are complex trade-offs between programmes that benefit the individual and those that benefit society. In approaches that are based on the best interest of the individual or on the public good, people are persuaded or forced to accept an intervention, overriding their autonomy. Programmes need to be based on respect for the autonomy of individuals and their rights. In programmes based on respect for the individual's autonomy, their capacity to understand and make their own decisions is respected and the health worker is an adviser, partner or facilitator (O'Keefe, 1995a). Given the equivocal benefit of much preventive medicine, it is important that the rights of individuals are respected, that they are informed of the benefits and risks, and that their decisions are respected.

Conclusions

Preventive programmes are taking over more areas of our lives. Ivan Illich (1975) sees these trends as leading to what he describes as 'social iatrogenesis', creating a situation where people are encouraged to see themselves as patients and to see medical care as the solution to their problems. Genetic testing promises whole new areas for intervention and vast potential markets. Toxic drugs, such as Tamoxifen, can be prescribed in order to prevent breast cancer and this could be a growing trend. David Armstrong (1995) has argued that the 'hospital model' of medical practice established in the nineteenth century, is being replaced by a 'surveillance' model. Illness used to be seen as temporary and confined to hospitals, where people gave up control to experts. Chronic or potential illness is now seen as the norm and, by implication, people give up control permanently. This is the surveillance model. Health promotion and preventive medicine, such as screening, changing attitudes and behaviour, changing the content of school curricula or banning smoking, all bring methods of control outside the hospital.

Health education, immunization and screening, do not usually empower individuals or communities, but encourage them to rely on the 'technical fix' and, incidentally, provide new markets for drugs, equipment and the health industries. Rosalind Coward, in discussing the growth of complementary and alternative approaches, summarizes some dangers in trends that see health as something within an individual's control:

> Does the active involvement of the individual in determining the course of their life have to be won by swallowing a moral code where blame attaches to the failure to be healthy in body and mind? Does a sense of control and responsibility have to be focused on internal transformations, and behaviour adjustments? Or are these, in fact, one way in which people will remain out of control of the major social decisions which affect their lives? (1989: 93)

4

RESEARCH

It's always the patient who has to take the chance when an experiment
is necessary. And we can find out nothing without experiment.

George Bernard Shaw *The Doctor's Dilemma* (1906)

Research should be undertaken with women and not on women.

Charter for Ethical Research in Maternity Care AIMS and NCT (1997)

We rely on researchers to increase our understanding of diseases and
develop more effective ways of treating them. In addition, achieving
efficiency and effectiveness – major preoccupations of Western health
policy – relies on research and audit to provide the evidence base for
clinical practice. Research needs patients, but in spite of this, in science-led
research, they are seen only as the host of the disease or the 'human
subjects'. In epidemiological research patients are only important for the
personal characteristics that make them statistically more, or less, likely to
develop a disease. Excluding users from research, except as its subjects,
has meant that much health research is irrelevant to the experiences of
patients and carers. Users can contribute in a number of ways. First, they
can ensure that their rights and those of other patients are observed and
they are protected from harm. Secondly, they need to help decide the
areas of research and audit, since research directions will influence the
future health services available to them. Thirdly, more user involvement
may help to improve the quality of research and ensure that there is more
public scrutiny of research. Finally, more user involvement may ensure
that the results of research and audit are used to improve health care.

Rights of participants

Research is undertaken to find out whether or not the drug or intervention
which is being tested will benefit patients and what side effects it may
have. In research into new drugs (phase I trials), the substance is first
tested on healthy people who volunteer – from altruism or for payment.

Then the substance will be tried out on a few patients to see if it is active against the disease in the short term (phase II trials). If it proves to be active, phase III trials are carried out on several hundred or several thousand patients, before it is licensed.

Since there is always the possibility of benefit or harm from participating in trials, informed consent is considered to be more important in research than in treatment; research ethics committees are required to ensure that research carried out on patients and healthy volunteers is ethical.

Informed consent

The concept of informed consent was part of the judgement at the Nuremberg trials when 23 German doctors were charged with carrying out medical research of such inhumanity as to constitute war crimes. This was followed up by the World Medical Association in the Declaration of Helsinki, which was first issued in 1964 and revised in 1975. Under the Helsinki Declaration, consent is not necessary if the physician considers that it is not essential to obtain informed consent. However, the specific reasons for this must be included in the protocol and approved by an independent committee.

Guidelines from the Royal College of Physicians (1996) state that patients have an absolute right to agree to participate in or to withdraw from trials at any time. However, there may be a conflict between the researchers' need to recruit subjects and the 'best interest' of patients. Researchers want to persuade patients to join and then continue in trials, while patients want to ensure there is something to be gained by them (or for future generations if they are motivated by altruism) from participating in the research. This conflict of interest is particularly evident where the researcher is also the clinician. GPs, for example, receive payment for recruiting their patients into drug trials and patients may feel that they cannot refuse to participate because of their ongoing relationship with the doctor. A review of randomized controlled trials on children found that consent rates were particularly high in trials on in-patients and newborn babies. This suggests that people find it particularly difficult to refuse to participate in trials when in hospital (Campbell et al., 1997). Refugees and asylum seekers may also be particularly vulnerable to pressures since, if refugee status is not granted, participation in medical trials is one reason that the Home Office may consider in appeals against deportation.

Some professionals are reluctant to accept the need for informed consent and argue that to forewarn a patient about the exact nature of the trial may distort the results and reduce its scientific value. Furthermore, it may be 'needlessly cruel' to give people more information than they may want and to ask them to make a difficult decision at a time when they may be feeling upset and confused (Tobias and Souhami, 1993). Another disadvantage is that if people have too much information and fully understand the nature of the research, they may see no benefit and will refuse to join trials. The requirement to obtain informed consent presents additional difficulties where research depends on large numbers. In the 1950s randomized controlled trials for drugs included tens of patients, by the 1960s it was hundreds, in the 1970s it had grown to thousands, and in the 1980s, it was tens of thousands. Now with even larger international studies, obtaining fully informed consent for such vast numbers is expensive.

To overcome the difficulties faced by researchers, it has been argued that patients should be asked to give their 'blanket consent' when they go into hospitals where randomized trials are being undertaken (Tobias, 1997; Brewin, 1997). Consent should be based, it is argued, on trust rather than information. Patients cannot, however, always assume their trust will be fulfilled. People in the UK have been included in trials without their knowledge or consent, sometimes with devastating consequences. RAGE (Radiotherapy Action Group Exposure) was set up by women who found out that they had received experimental radiotherapy treatment for cervical cancer. Because of the treatment they had serious internal damage, sometimes requiring a colostomy. One woman died as a result of the treatment. Another woman describes how, when six months after treatment she returned to the hospital with severe faecal incontinence, she was told that she might have radiotherapy damage and was 'unlucky'. Only later did she realize that there were many other 'unlucky' women who were also badly damaged and that hundreds of women had been involved in clinical trials of radiotherapy to the pelvic area. None had been informed that they were in a clinical trial (RAGE National, 1997).

As regulation tightens up and researchers are more restricted in what they can do, trials may be carried out on people in disadvantaged communities and developing countries. In 1997 there was controversy about HIV research trials in developing countries. Studies in the USA and France showed that it was possible to reduce the rate of HIV transmission from mother to baby if the mother took zidovudine (AZT) from mid-pregnancy. Studies were then undertaken in African countries to try a lower dosage than that used in the trials in the USA and France, and to compare this with a placebo. Critics said this was unethical because some women would not receive treatment that was known to reduce the chance of their baby being born HIV positive. The lower dosage, they argued, should have been compared with the higher doses given in the West (Angell, 1997). The researchers defended their position by arguing that health care was such in the countries concerned that the women who participated would not have received the drugs anyway. Poorer and disadvantaged people will, on these arguments, always be available as subjects for research which would be unethical if undertaken on better-off people. This excuse was used to defend the Tuskegee syphilis study. This study lasted from 1932 to 1972 and took place in one of the poorest counties of Alabama. It followed the natural history of syphilis in four hundred untreated African-Americans. Elaborate steps were taken to ensure that the survivors remained untreated, even after the introduction of penicillin.

Randomized controlled trials

Randomized controlled trials are an efficient and impartial way of finding out about the impact of a treatment or intervention. They are considered to be the gold standard of medical research. Patients in the trial are assigned randomly to different treatment groups and, ideally, neither patient nor clinician knows which regime patients are receiving, since if they do, this can bias the results.

However, randomized controlled trials are not suited to all clinical research and may sometimes cost too much – in human and ethical terms. First, in the interests of research some patients are given the new treatment and some are not. Patients are asked to give up their right to choose what treatment they receive, since they will be randomly allocated to different treatment groups. Many patients find it distressing to give up their choice and lose control.

Secondly, if clinicians are convinced of the benefit of a particular treatment, undertaking research which involves one group of patients receiving a placebo may be unethical. Patients and doctors often believe, sometimes rightly and sometimes wrongly, in the benefits of the new treatment on trial. In such trials it is distressing for patients who believe that they are receiving the placebo and not the 'best' treatment available. To doctors it may appear unethical to withhold the new treatment from any of their patients. Sometimes a trial is stopped early because the initial results are good, without waiting to see whether any long-term problems emerge. This happened with the trials for AZT and for hormone replacement therapy (HRT). It was only after the drugs were licensed and longer trials carried out that AZT proved to be ineffective by itself and the possible links between HRT and cancer emerged.

Thirdly, randomized controlled trials are difficult to use in some areas of research, such as the estimation of the effect of treatments on the quality of life. It is also difficult with randomized controlled trials to evaluate interventions such as surgery, psychiatry or complementary therapies, where success depends on the skills of the practitioner, and on the attitudes and personalities of patients and clinicians. In addition, some complementary practitioners also have ethical problems in participating in randomized controlled trials that compare their treatments with orthodox ones. For example, the Bristol Cancer Help Centre started in 1980 as a small self-help group to help people cope with cancer, using diet, nutrition, relaxation and meditation. It was willing to participate in research, but was not willing to refuse help to people who came to the Centre by entering them into a control group in a trial.

Some of the problems of informed consent and randomized controlled trials can be illustrated by the large-scale investigation of breast cancer carried out between 1980 and 1985. This trial involved 2230 women in 30 hospitals, and included looking at the impact on women of offering support and counselling after treatment. One group was given counselling and one group was not. Initially the local research ethics committee, which was responsible for approving the research, had insisted that informed consent must be obtained. Consequently women were asked if they would participate in the trial when they arrived at the hospital for an operation. This caused the women so much distress that, rather than insist that researchers must ask women before admission and give them time to think about it, the ethics committee withdrew their stipulation for informed consent (Faulder, 1985). Women were not informed that they were participating in a randomized trial. The situation came to light when one unwitting participant, Evelyn Thomas, realized that she had been involved in the trial when she read about the research findings. She then understood why, shortly after the operation, the woman in the next bed who had been through a similar operation was treated differently to her. Her neighbour received counselling and was given useful information. The counsellor, she said, 'avoided me and a breast prosthesis was given to me by a male fitter more used to fitting artificial limbs' (Walker, 1993: 327).

Relevant information at an appropriate time is necessary to ensure that patients can give informed consent. The timing of the approach by the investigator is important. Sometimes people who have just been given a diagnosis are in a state of shock and may not be aware of the significance of what they are being asked to do or the risks that they may be taking. This is not a good time to ask them to make a decision. People need information in language that is easy to understand, time to think about the implications of participating and to talk with people they are close to.

Research ethics committees

The Helsinki Declaration on ethics and research recommended in 1964 that research ethics committees should be set up. In 1967 the Royal College of Physicians first recommended that every institution that undertook clinical research should have a group of doctors to satisfy itself of the ethics of a proposed investigation. In 1975 the Department of Health and Social Security advised district health authorities to set up research ethics committees to review all research projects. The purpose of the committees was to maintain high ethical standards in the conduct of clinical research and to ensure that procedures did not endanger the safety or well-being of subjects.

There is widespread criticism of ethics committees (Meade, 1994; Harries et al., 1994). A study undertaken by Rabbi Julia Neuberger in 1992 noted that local research ethics committees had been set up in a haphazard way and that their membership and the way they operated varied enormously. Though there were guidelines from the Department of Health, many committees did not follow them. Committees were dominated by hospital doctors, 44 per cent did not include a pharmacist or clinical pharmacologist as a member, even though most of the research they vetted involved drugs. In some areas not all research was submitted to the ethics committee. In general, research committees were overloaded with proposals, leading to delays. Many did not monitor projects to see if their recommendations had been followed.

Committees consider many issues that are not just scientific and medical, but of public concern. Lawyers, clergy and moral philosophers as well as users have a contribution to make to their work. In spite of Department of Health guidelines (1991b) which recommend that ethics committees should have at least two lay members, one third of committees had fewer than two lay members. There were few women and even fewer members from minority ethnic communities on research ethics committees (Neuberger, 1992).

Though one of the aims of research ethics committees is to promote public confidence in research, they do not work in an open way. Proceedings are often confidential which is necessary, it is claimed, to ensure that rival researchers do not find out about developments or products. Secrecy about research may be occasionally justified for commercial reasons, but it cannot be argued that it is for the benefit of patients. Furthermore, confidentiality creates difficulties for 'lay' members who are not able to ask advice from anyone outside the committee. 'Lay' people on professional committees may feel that their expertise is not recognized or appreciated and they often feel marginalized. This is partly because the duties and accountability of 'lay' members have never been clearly defined.

Multi-centre trials have to be approved by ethics committees in each participating centre. The varied responses to identical applications showed just how differently committees viewed the same research proposal. As a result, regional committees were set up in 1997 to advise on multi-centre trials. Some of the differences in local research ethics committees are due to lack of guidance or local diversity, but others may depend on the moral outlook of the research ethics committee itself (Foster, 1995). If members are committed primarily to the value of research, they may not consider informed consent to be so important. If they look at research from the perspective of patients' rights, the support of users and user groups is important. Thus one committee may see informed consent as essential, whereas others may feel that in research sometimes the ends justify the means. There is a need for a national framework to help members of local committees assess difficult moral questions, such as research on children, people with mental health problems or who are confused as well as healthy volunteers who receive payment.

Research ethics committees are important since they are the only regulatory point through which all proposed clinical research is likely to pass and their role needs to be extended. First, the membership needs to be strengthened and the status of lay members raised. This requires that members are appointed in an open way and have the skills needed to assess research and safeguard patients. In Denmark, half the members of research ethics committees are lay people, chosen by the county council rather than the health service.

Secondly, ethics committees could influence the quality of research undertaken in their area. Research ethics committees could take a more proactive role and, for example, require systematic reviews of existing research to make sure that the research is needed before they approve a new proposal. Some commentators have suggested that research committees may be behaving unethically by endorsing new research that is unnecessary and by acquiescing in the failure of researchers to publish research which does not give the desired results. Savulescu and colleagues (1996) have suggested that ethics committees should be made accountable for poor research.

Thirdly, they could strengthen the position of users in research by insisting, for example, that participants in research know the reasons for the research, its potential significance as well as its potential harm, and its source of funding as conditions of approval. They could also insist that research results are made publicly accessible.

Finally, local ethics committees could encourage research that reflects the priorities of the health service, users and the needs of the local population. They could advise health authorities and providers on the nature of the research being undertaken and areas where they feel research is most needed.

Research directions

The research topics of today determine the treatments and services that will be available tomorrow. For example, if research concentrates on the development of new drugs to relieve pain, rather than other pain relieving techniques, the chances are that these drugs will be offered to patients in the future. Some areas, such as mental illness and learning difficulties, have been poorly researched. This reflects and maintains the low priority and limited resources given to providing services for people with learning difficulties and mental health problems.

Medical research tends to concentrate on narrow science-based questions that do not take account of the subjective views of users. A survey of health service research, excluding pharmaceutical research, found that most studies looked at specific diseases or assessed health technologies and equipment. Conditions that caused severe discomfort, but were not life-threatening, were poorly represented (Dowie, 1995). This trend is reflected elsewhere. In India a survey of research published between 1987 and 1994 found that most medical research was about tertiary health care and the new biology – and irrelevant to the country's major health problems (Mudur, 1997).

The source of funding dominates the overall direction of medical research. Funding comes from the government, charitable foundations and commercial interests. According to the Association of Medical Research Charities, in 1992–93, 56.3 per cent of health research and development was funded by the pharmaceutical industry, 12.9 per cent by medical charities, 10.2 per cent by the NHS, 9.3 per cent by the universities, 8.1 per cent by the Medical Research Council and 2.7 per cent by the Department of Health. Government funding for research is important because it is more likely to look at innovative approaches that may lead to reductions in costs and in the use of drugs. However, it has decreased since 1980, making researchers more dependent on commercial funding.

The public contributes to research through donations to medical charities: in 1996–97 the big research charities in the Association of Medical Research Charities spent £420 million on medical research. Charitable funds tend to look at specific diseases and concentrate on acute specialties. Within medical research charities, cancer and leukaemia received 39 per cent of expenditure, compared to 2.6 per cent on neurology and mental health. The public tend to give money to a cause – such as the search for a 'cure' for cancer or the latest diagnostic equipment – without necessarily understanding that the money may not achieve what they hope. 'Cures' for cancer have proved elusive and often diagnostic equipment is initially more useful for research and only much later improves treatment.

Users of specific services may differ from professionals in their priorities for research and may want different outcomes (Williamson, 1992). For example, most cancer trials are about chemotherapy. However, one survey found that women with breast cancer wanted more research on the impact of treatments on their quality of life, environmental issues, psychosocial issues and the optimum dose of radiotherapy required to control the tumour while at the same time causing minimum damage to healthy tissues (Goodare and Smith, 1995). Similarly, most research around childbirth is focused on the effectiveness of drugs and interventions. Members of the National Childbirth Trust wanted more research into effective communication and support to meet individual parents' needs (Oliver, 1995).

Decisions about how the main medical charities spend their money are determined by professionals, in their positions as members of scientific advisory panels. These panels make decisions about which research to fund and tend to support orthodox approaches. These panels do not normally include lay members or people who have the condition, whose opinions may widen their discussions. Trustees of the charities do not make the decisions for themselves because, according to a leaflet from the Association of Medical Research Charities: 'Lay trustees may not fully understand scientific research proposals and, without expert advice, the funding decision may be based only on the persuasiveness of the scientists, how many trustees they know or are able to influence, or how much money they can control for themselves'. However, professional members may be even more open to these influences than users or 'lay' people. A study in Sweden found that peer reviewers could not judge scientific merit independently of gender and comradeship. Women fared poorly and researchers with whom reviewers were affiliated did better (Wenneras and Wold, 1997). Lay trustees, in contrast, are primarily interested in practical outcomes of research that benefit the people for whom the charity was set up.

Some user groups are now questioning whether experts have the right approach to research questions after all. Researchers do not usually live day-to-day with the condition that is the area of their research; many treat only a few patients and do not meet their carers. The Insulin Dependent Diabetes Trust (IDDT) point out how easy it would be for users to regain control of the money that they now hand over to professionals.

> The whole issue could be turned on its head. All charities, like the IDDT, have a Board of Trustees and usually the vast majority of these elected Trustees are non-medical. It is surely this body that should not only decide on how much of this money is spent on research but should also decide the direction of research. In other words they should divide up the pot of money into various categories they want researched and then invite applications from researchers. The role of the experts would then be in deciding on whether the applications are scientifically and methodologically correct. (IDDT, 1997a)

According to the Pharmaceutical Industry Council (1997), UK drug companies spend more than £3 billion a year on research, though other estimates are lower at just over £2 billion (Consumers' Association et al., 1997). With the decline in public funding for research, the amount of research funded by drug companies has increased and the pharmaceutical industry is now the chief funder of research. Pharmaceutical company research is subsidized, intentionally but indirectly, by the profit margins allowed by the Department of Health through the Pharmaceutical Price Regulation Scheme. This is a voluntary agreement between the Department of Health and the Association of the British Pharmaceutical Industry which was introduced in 1969. Companies negotiate target profits from sales to the NHS at 17–21 per cent as the rate of return on their investment in research and development. They set their own prices and can negotiate increases to achieve the target rate of return if they forecast that profits will be less than 75 per cent of their target. The Scheme has been criticized because it operates in secrecy, with little accountability or involvement of users or health professionals (Earl-Slater, 1997). Though the scheme was set up in 1969, the first annual report was only published 27 years later in 1996.

Subsidizing drug research through the Pharmaceutical Price Regulation Scheme means that the government, professionals and users have no influence on research carried out. Drug companies fund research that meets the needs of the industry, which may not be the same as the needs of patients or the NHS. For drug companies the most profitable research may be into 'me-too' drugs, which are variations on other companies' or even their own drugs. For example, 13 per cent of all drugs approved by the US Food and Drug Administration before 1990 were rated A (important therapeutic gain over currently marketed drugs); 37 per cent were rated B (moderate therapeutic gain) and 50 per cent were rated C (little or no therapeutic gain) (Bero and Rennie, 1996). Research into new drugs for specific high profile conditions, such as HIV and AIDS, can also be profitable – especially where users can be relied on to press for the drugs to be licensed more quickly than normal and, once licensed, to be prescribed widely. There is little research on drugs for tropical diseases, such as malaria, where there is a great need but the market is poor.

Commercially funded research is also concerned with treating symptoms – not with understanding the disease process or the interaction of the individual and the environment with the disease. Prevention is only of interest if it involves early diagnosis and so provides the opportunity to develop new treatments and new markets. For example, although the causes of asthma have not been accurately pinpointed, they are recognized to be in the environment. However, the main response has been to improve the management of asthma by the use of drugs. Treatments for asthma are effective, at least in the short term: salbutamol can be used to deal with the immediate symptoms of an attack by relaxing the muscles in spasm, whereas steroids taken regularly can deal with inflammation and improve general lung function. However, there are limitations in the long term to these treatments, which only address symptoms and not the causes of asthma attacks. Research suggests that the introduction of adrenalin sprays in the treatment of asthma may have caused a sudden increase in asthma deaths from 1948 (Blauw and Westendorp, 1995). There have been increases in deaths when some other new asthma drugs have been introduced. In New Zealand the epidemic of deaths following the introduction of Fenterol continued to be high for a decade. The reasons for these disturbing patterns are not clear, but point to the importance of funding research into prevention, and non-drug treatments and management.

Many researchers have a vested interest in ill health and its treatment through drugs and surgery rather than other approaches, such as nutrition, which involve little technology and may cost less. The pharmaceutical industry has little incentive to fund the sort of research that is of most use to the practitioner – cheaper, off-patent or non-drug alternatives.

Designing research

Though research design and methods are seen as technical and professional matters, the way participants behave affects the quality of research. In research trials as well as in clinical practice, patients may not comply with instructions, often without the researchers' knowledge, and so distort the research results. This is known to have happened in US research trials for AZT. Some patients had their prescribed pills tested to see if they were receiving AZT or the placebo. If the pills were placebos, some then obtained AZT on the black market or shared out their AZT outside the clinic. If people understand why research is being carried out before they agree to participate, they may be more likely to comply with instructions and continue in trials.

Greater user involvement in the design of trials may also prevent the halting of expensive trials. The National Women's Health Network managed to stop a large trial on the use of Tamoxifen to prevent breast cancer, run by the National Institute of Health in the USA. They discovered that the trial's organizers had been associated with irregular research and were accused in Congress of delaying the publication of results that showed that Tamoxifen was associated with endometrial cancer. If women with long experience of the side effects of Tamoxifen had been consulted the US trial might have been designed differently or never started (Goodare and Smith, 1995). In Britain, the Medical Research Council withdrew its support for a similar trial after a controversial debate and public pressure, because of concerns about the toxicity of Tamoxifen. The trial took place, funded by medical charities.

Poor research design can cause great distress to participants, as illustrated by the Bristol cancer research trials. Although most people attending the Bristol Cancer Help Centre had had orthodox treatment for their cancer, the medical establishment was hostile to the Centre. The Centre, confident in its work, agreed to a three-year-study of its patients involving quantitative and qualitative research by the Imperial Cancer Research Fund. However, interim results were published at a major press conference after only 18 months. These concluded that women, who were at the time of their attendance at Bristol free of relapse, were almost three times more likely to relapse than those who did not attend the Bristol Centre. Press headlines claimed 'Cancer spread is likelier with holistic therapy'. Even the *British Medical Journal* ran the headline: 'Death from complementary therapy'. The results seemed to be a resounding triumph for orthodox cancer therapies.

It was soon clear that the research was flawed and the findings did not support the claims of the interim report. However, enormous damage had been done to the Centre. The Bristol Survey Support Group was set up to help those who felt that they had been abused by the survey. Participants were very distressed to be told that they were more likely to die because they had been to the Centre and felt that they had been misled by the researchers who seemed only to want to support their own prejudices and had dropped the qualitative aspects of the research (Goodare, 1996). One of the eminent researchers committed suicide following the controversy.

Greater user involvement in the design of trials may improve the quality of the research and make it more acceptable to participants. One study used focus groups, with members recruited through a local cancer support group, to find out patients' views of a protocol for a clinical trial. The group identified a number of factors which might make patients reluctant to co-operate. As a result changes were made to the protocol. The study concluded that using focus groups to find out patients' perceptions at an initial stage may save time and money, increase participation levels and lead to better results (Bradburn et al., 1995).

Research methods

Some drugs seem to give good results in trials but prove dangerous or ineffective after long-term use. Bero and Rennie (1996) concluded that research was often flawed by the most basic errors in design and analysis. Sometimes, in order to produce the desired results, researchers failed to randomize subjects properly, removed data, and also divided their data into smaller sub-groups. They chose narrow research questions and looked at the effectiveness, but not the toxicity, of a drug. They used higher dosages in comparative trials so that their drugs appeared more effective than other drugs that were already on the market. New drugs were compared in trials with a placebo rather than other drugs on the market. Research carried out in this way gives biased results, but the results can be profitably used in marketing by the pharmaceutical company.

Patients included in trials are often not representative of the people who are likely to be given the drug once it has been licensed. Clinical trials are conducted by specialists on selected patients who are usually in hospital and suffering from a precisely diagnosed condition. In trials patients are given drugs at the right dose and at the right time, after ensuring that they are not taking any other medication which might interact with the drug being tested. Women of childbearing age are often excluded from trials, to protect the foetus and avoid potential litigation in case they are pregnant. Although half of new cancers emerge in people over 70, cancer in the elderly is poorly treated and poorly understood because elderly people are often excluded from clinical cancer trials (Fentimen et al., 1990). For good reasons, children too are often excluded from research trials – not least because they are not able to give their informed consent to participate in research in which they may risk harm as well as benefit.

In the real world these conditions do not often apply. Once a drug is licensed there will be forceful marketing to persuade GPs and other clinicians to prescribe it for a variety of conditions, including to women of childbearing age, children and older people. This is an important issue. For example, a survey found that a quarter of children in hospital were given drugs that were unlicensed for use in children or were prescribed outside the terms of the product licence (Turner et al., 1998). Problems also arose for elderly people with the anti-arthritis drug Opren. Although the clinical trial for the drug included patients over the age of 65, they were not followed up to see the way that different doses worked in older people. In older people the drug took much longer to clear from their systems and this led eventually to a build-up and physiological damage. In the 1980s over four thousand people, many of them elderly, contacted the Opren Action Group alleging some injury; a further number, about one hundred, had died.

Measuring successful outcomes

Patients cannot make informed choices about treatment without knowing about the likely success and side effects of different treatments as well as what is likely to happen if they have no treatment at all. The criteria chosen to assess the effectiveness of treatments are, therefore, very important. Professionals, not patients, have defined what factors are measured as 'outcomes' for treatment. For example, length of survival is the traditional measure of success for many treatments, but this does not take account of the quality of the remaining life. Sometimes, a good outcome of treatment for cancer may be prolonged life and for patients, carers and professionals to feel that they have tried everything. Sometimes, however, the pain and disability may not be worth the struggle to the patient and a good outcome is a dignified and quicker death. Patients, carers and professionals may each have different views of what is a good outcome of treatment and assess the quality of life after treatment differently (Frater, 1992).

Sometimes surrogate (or substitute) outcome measures are used which may not relate to a 'cure' or be relevant to the actual experiences of patients. For example, new cancer drugs do not always have to demonstrate that they lengthen the life of people with cancer or improve their quality of life as long as they shrink tumours. Similarly, in anorexia nervosa, weight gain and, for women, menstruation are the most commonly used measures in research studies. However, weight may not be a good measure in the long term; it has been noted that people who are forced to eat often lose weight again as soon as they are out of hospital. For some people with anorexia nervosa it is enough that they maintain a viable weight, though this may be well below what is generally seen as 'normal' (Halek, 1994).

Another example of surrogate outcome measures is in childbirth research which often monitors the outcome of an intervention for babies, but not for mothers – whether it is of infection rates or side effects of drugs. Similarly, trials looking into the effects of social support for disadvantaged mothers evaluate how women feel physically and emotionally and how they cope socially. However, the outcome measures used in evaluating strategies for helping pregnant women to give up smoking tend to be obstetric ones: such as birthweight and perinatal mortality. Since smoking is a way that women cope with stress, it seems irrational to eradicate a coping mechanism and not assess any of the social and emotional consequences of doing this (Oliver, 1997). Sometimes obvious outcomes are not measured. It would be easy, for example, to see if people on psychiatric drugs are less likely to commit suicide. It is odd that there is no published evidence that antidepressants are helpful in reducing suicide. In fact one study showed an increased suicide rate, perhaps partly because antidepressants are drugs commonly used in suicides (Breggin, 1993).

The quality of life a treatment offers is an important consideration for users. Economists have developed QALYs (Quality-Adjusted Life Years) as a tool to assess the cost–benefit of particular treatments. Each treatment is measured in terms of how many years of life the recipient of the treatment can expect and the quality of life it will give. This approach was criticized since it was based on limited research into how patients and carers assessed quality of life. In addition, it replaced the belief that everyone had an equal right to health care with the belief that people should be selected according to particular characteristics, which raises ethical problems in deciding who 'deserves' treatment and why. Economists may be offering a technical solution to what is essentially a political problem (Carr Hill, 1991).

In measuring outcomes it is often important to take a long-term view. The funders of research tend to look for short-term results, though the real outcome for the patient may not be clear until years after treatment. The lack of long-term research means that actual death and complication rates are not known or are underestimated. For example, Spiegal and colleagues (1989) found that support groups for women with advanced breast cancer and their families could alleviate some of the stresses they faced, but had not affected the length of their survival after 18 months. Little notice was taken of this research until researchers followed up the women after ten years to see what had happened to them, with the intention of debunking the theory that an improved emotional state would affect the course of the disease (Batt, 1994). Though 83 of the 86 women had died, those in the treatment group had lived an average of 18 months longer than the control group. It is also disquieting to note that side effects can be passed down the generations. In the 1940s, stilboestrol was given to pregnant women to prevent miscarriage. Over twenty years later children developed cancers and other problems as a result.

Drugs which may be used long term are sometimes licensed on the basis of short-term results. One example is Xanax which is a minor tranquillizer that is widely used in the USA to treat panic attacks but is not available on the NHS. It was introduced after an eight-week study but marketing and advertising of the drug only included the results up to four weeks. After eight weeks the patients receiving a placebo were doing as well as the patients on Xanax. However, in the long term, patients taking placebos were better off because Xanax is highly addictive and they did not suffer the severe withdrawal and rebound reactions of those taking the drug. People on Xanax experienced an increase in anxiety and phobic responses – and a 350 per cent greater number of panic attacks when they came off the drug (Breggin, 1993). More recently Prozac was licensed in the USA based on scientifically controlled trials that lasted five and six weeks and it is still not known if it is addictive.

The Medicines Control Agency, which is responsible for licensing new drugs, is not always proactive in checking safety after the licensing. It was many years before the addictive qualities of benzodiazepines, such as Valium, Librium and Xanax, were recognized. For example, in 1980 the Medicines Control Agency concluded that benzodiazepine tranquillizers rarely caused dependence, whereas five years later, the estimates were that between a quarter and half million people in the UK were affected by benzodiazepine dependency (Medewar, 1992). The problem with drugs that create dependence is that withdrawal symptoms may be confused with recurrence of symptoms of the condition that was originally being treated. If someone has withdrawal symptoms, therefore, this may seem to be evidence of the effectiveness of the drug in suppressing symptoms. There are suggestions that dependence problems are arising with the group of SSRI antidepressants – which includes Prozac (Medewar, 1997).

Despite the methodological difficulties that exist, patients and carers need to be involved in defining and assessing outcomes. This requires a range of different techniques, both qualitative and quantitative. In order to decide what outcomes to measure, researchers need to start with what is the purpose of treatment, what the patient's problems are, what other options are open to them, and what are the potential risks and benefits of therapy (Coulter, 1994).

Publication of research

Increasingly research funding is by pharmaceutical companies, who are interested in results that favour their product and who want secrecy to prevent competitors knowing about any developments or breakthroughs. Often a condition of drug company funding is that the results cannot be published without their permission. As a result researchers may be prevented from publishing unwanted, generally unfavourable, research results. In one instance there was a seven-year delay in publishing a study comparing a brand drug with a generic drug because it showed that the brand drug, which was more expensive, was no better than the generic equivalent (Wise, 1997). Secrecy means that knowledge is not readily shared in the research community and it is easier to cover up poor results and even make up false ones. The amount of fraud in medical research is increasing (Lock and Wells, 1996). The stakes are high in drug trials and it is increasingly difficult to check results because computer data and digital imaging can be edited in a way that raw data in notebooks could not be.

As a result, studies that do not have significant results (though this may in itself be significant) or that produce results which do not fit into received wisdom may have difficulty in obtaining further funding and may go unreported. As scientific consensus is often reached by a synthesis of all published reports, under-reporting of results may lead to misleading conclusions. If research is relevant and properly conducted, the results are important – even if they seem boring or improbable or do not fit into the marketing strategy of the funders (Pearn, 1995).

Individual participants should have the right to information about research in which they have participated and, in randomized controlled trials, to know whether they received the placebo or the treatment being tested. They should be informed of the results before publication. However, this often does not happen because editors of medical journals fear that results will leak out and appear in the mass media before they appear in journals (Lowry and Smith, 1992). In occupational health research, results are announced to participants before publication, giving those people affected directly by the research an opportunity to question researchers. This is far better, for example, than hearing on the TV news that your children have an increased chance of developing leukaemia. The meeting between researchers and workers usually takes place early in the week of publication. This arrangement could be followed for the results of other research (Goodare and Smith, 1995).

Improving health care

Research knowledge, however important, is often slow to reach practitioners. The Parliamentary Select Committee on Medical Research in 1988 found that medical research was poorly resourced, morale was low, and that the NHS had been run with little awareness of the needs of research or what it had to offer. Research findings may take a long time to influence clinical practice because of the deep-seated professional reluctance to question established practice or to use the results of research to criticize, even implicitly, the clinical judgement of colleagues.

The separation of research and clinical practice sometimes means that procedures which are known to be ineffective or even to be harmful are still widely used. This is a very old problem. In 1938 Dr J.A. Glover demonstrated that children in Peterborough were ten times more likely to have their tonsils removed than children in Hornsey, Wood Green or Finchley. Tonsillectomies became very fashionable and by the 1950s whole classes of school children in the Black country were admitted for the operation. Tonsillectomies are now considered to be 'discretionary' operations because the indications for doing them are not clear, but they are still the most common ENT operation and, what is more, there are still geographical variations. John Yates (1995) found that almost sixty years later Peterborough still had one of the highest rates in the country for admitting children with tonsillitis.

It was to address some of these problems that the NHS research and development (R&D) programme was set up in 1991 to promote and fund more applied research and promote greater clinical effectiveness in the NHS. The Department of Health set up a Clinical Outcomes Group, with a consumer sub-group to provide information on how to encourage and facilitate consumer involvement at national, regional and local level.

Clinical audit and improving practice

Clinical audit is the main mechanism to changing practice. Clinical audit, introduced in the 1980s, is based on peer review to support staff to improve their performance rather than to penalize them. Clinical audit is generally confidential – otherwise clinicians might not co-operate or give information that reveals their shortcomings. For example, consultants who participated in the National Confidential Enquiry into Perioperative Deaths were not identified and data were destroyed before publication so that clinicians, patients, hospitals and districts could not be identified retrospectively (Buck et al., 1989). Some confidentiality may be necessary in audit, but information about standards of individual practitioners is important for managers to ensure that patients are not put at risk. Safeguards are needed so that the duty of confidentiality to the practitioner is not seen as more important than the duty to protect patients.

Clinical audit is often seen as a professional matter where users have little to contribute. There has been resistance from some audit committees to the involvement of 'outsiders', including managers and other professionals, on the grounds of protecting patient confidentiality (Buttery et al., 1994). The involvement of users at local level has so far been patchy and limited (Kelson, 1995; Joule, 1992). Users' views may be dismissed as uninformed or erroneous. The views of patients tend to be sought for interpersonal and organizational aspects of care, but it is assumed that they cannot assess clinical competence.

Obstacles can be overcome if there is a will to involve users. A study in Newcastle showed a variety of ways that mental health service users could be involved in clinical audit (Balogh and Bond, 1995). In some areas open-ended group discussions were held with current and past users to identify topics for audit; in others, representatives, who had themselves used mental health services, were included as core members of the audit team. In another area, users currently receiving care were invited to participate in workshops. This was seen as a valuable way of ensuring that users' perspectives were kept to the fore. However, there were some difficulties if the user was discharged during the audit or if staff involved in their care were also on the audit team.

Research and changing practice

The difficulties in putting research findings into practice should not be underestimated. For example, childbirth is one area where Department of

Health policy changed in the 1990s on the basis of research evidence, but practice has not yet changed in line with this. Before 1948 most babies were delivered at home by a midwife. With the advent of the NHS, a birth in hospital and a doctor in attendance became available to everyone. This changed the whole experience of childbirth. Whereas midwives tended to believe in watching and waiting, doctors preferred to take control of labour. New maternity units were set up and home midwifery services were run down. In 1960 30 per cent of all births took place at home, in 1970 this dropped to 11 per cent and in 1985 to less than 1 per cent. By 1995 it had increased slightly but was still less than 2 per cent of all births (Office for National Statistics, 1997). Gradually, women who wanted a home birth with a midwife came to be seen as irrational and almost deviant.

Interventions in labour and childbirth such as episiotomies, continuous foetal monitoring, forceps deliveries, induced labour and epidurals became common. As the Audit Commission (1997) recognized, one intervention can lead to another. For example, routine continuous electronic foetal monitoring and epidural analgesia increase the likelihood of a subsequent forceps or Caesarean delivery. In 1953, 2.2 per cent of births involved Caesarean sections; by 1978 this had increased to 7.3 per cent (McFarlane and Mugford, 1992). Since then the Caesarean section rate has increased sharply and a report by the Audit Commission in 1997 found the rates varied between 11 and 18 per cent in different hospitals. High intervention rates also became a part of defensive obstetrics: doctors were less likely to be sued if things went wrong if they had intervened than if they had not.

However, the evidence did not support these interventions. In Oxford the Cochrane Centre undertook a systematic review of the effects of care during pregnancy and childbirth, resulting in a database that is continually updated. This review found that women who have elective Caesarean sections (that is without a medical reason) are between two and four times more likely to die than those who have a vaginal delivery (Enkin et al., 1992). Furthermore, most women who have Caesarean deliveries are less satisfied with their care, feel less supported and suffer increased post-natal ill-health, not to mention the additional costs to the health service (Audit Commission, 1997).

In 1993 an expert report for the Department of Health, *Changing Childbirth*, proposed changes to maternity services which would mean that each woman would have more choice and control over her labour and delivery: in where she gives birth, how she gives birth, in the pain relief used and who is with her during labour. However, changes in local services have been slow and there is no evidence that interventions in childbirth have decreased. Some of the initial support for the policy may have been that a midwifery-led service would be cheaper than a consultant-led one. However, continuity of care and better and safe services in the community are not cheap options. The implementation of *Changing Childbirth* has focused on the importance of a woman's right to choose and not so much on the safety and use of technology and interventions in labour.

Introducing new drugs

Though the introduction of many research findings into clinical practice may be slow, the introduction of new drugs is an exception. There is often pressure from professionals, commercial interests and users to make the newest drugs available as soon as possible. Once the rumour circulates that a new drug or a new treatment may soon be available, some users may demand it, leading to political pressure which may override the lack of evidence of its effectiveness, its side effects or possible long-term problems.

The introduction of human insulin is an example of a new drug approved after limited research. There are about 350 000 diabetics in the UK who are dependent on insulin, which, since its discovery in the 1920s until the early 1980s, was derived from animals. In 1982 genetically produced so-called 'human' insulin became available. 'Human' insulin was licensed and on the market in 1982, two years after the first study was published. There were no large scale trials carried out, even though problems are not likely to emerge in studies with twenty, thirty or fifty participants. By the late 1980s, 84 per cent of all people with diabetes had been transferred to 'human' insulin. However, there was no formal post-marketing surveillance and people started to complain of problems – coma caused by low blood sugar without the usual warning signs, memory loss, confusion, depression, joint pains and weight gain. Initially professionals did not believe that the problems reported by diabetics were due to the change in insulin and thought they were psychological (Hirst, 1997). There may sometimes be advantages in licensing some drugs quickly. However, the problems that users experience in having side effects of drugs recognized and taken seriously is important and indicates the need for strong post-marketing regulation that involves users.

Conclusions

Increasingly, user representatives are being asked to comment on the information to be given to patients to obtain informed consent, but they need to be involved at all stages to ensure the research is ethical. Without wider involvement there is a danger that user involvement will just make unethical research more acceptable. There are several reasons why users need to be involved as partners in research and not just as guinea pigs.

First, more user involvement may reduce the amount of unnecessary research. Looking at research from the point of view of users will clarify the reasons for undertaking the research. Some research is of benefit to commercial interests, some may be undertaken by academic departments or GPs in order to generate income; some research may benefit the career of the researchers, some may benefit patients; some research may not benefit the patient who participates but may benefit others in the future. Who is benefiting from research needs to be explicitly acknowledged so that people may make informed decisions on whether to participate. For example, patients may be unwilling to participate in research that compares a new drug with a placebo when the crucial question is whether the new drug is better than existing treatments (Koopmans, 1995).

Secondly, where patients and carers are involved in determining the topics for research, it is likely to be on areas that will make a difference to them and will give useful results. Users are likely to give more weight to long-term follow-ups of the quality of their lives after treatment. There need to be clear research strategies, at national and local levels, to encourage research that reflects the priorities of the health service, users and the needs of the local population.

Thirdly, the involvement of users may lead to the development of more appropriate research methods. Though randomized controlled trials are seen as the ideal, they have ethical and practical limitations. Information about many treatments and areas of health care is needed which they cannot explore. A range of methods are needed to give a more holistic view of the impact of treatment, in particular in qualitative research that values the subjective experiences of patients and carers. Research methods themselves can be used to help to empower users. Questionnaires using tick boxes may be easy to fill in and analyse but do not give people an opportunity to express their views and experiences or to come to a better understanding themselves through participating in research.

Finally, if information from all research is widely available, patients, carers and user groups are more likely to campaign for results to be implemented. The involvement of users may open up research to public scrutiny and increase accountability. This is important to counterbalance the drug companies who can manipulate user groups to promote their products and speed up the licensing process, before the long-term effects are known.

Rather than contributing to the development of evidence-based medicine, some trends in research may lead to escalating costs with little benefit to health – and may even put patients at risk. Many problems are caused by the lack of independent funding for research and increasing dependence on drug company funding. There is also a lack of public scrutiny which may mean that the implications and long-term consequences for the health service of the reduction in independent funding for research have not yet been fully recognized.

PART II
USERS AND CITIZENS

5

COMMUNITIES

The first step to democracy . . . is a ramp.

SCOPE, advertisement in *Campaign News*, (1997)

Many of the improvements that users want in health care cannot be tackled by an individual, but require collective action. These include decisions about what services are provided, how they are provided and to whom. How do users and citizens influence these decisions? Though there is no tradition in the NHS of democratic accountability or participation, managers have gradually taken on board that they need to consult local people and find out the views of 'customers' in order to make sure services are appropriate and acceptable to them. While the NHS employs a wide range of consultation techniques, including postal surveys, public meetings, focus groups and opinion polls, none enable members of the public to define the aims of the exercise or the methods involved (Cooper et al., 1995). However, new ways of involving communities are being developed as a way of tackling inequalities in health. The different approaches that have been used to involve users in planning and monitoring local services are explored in this chapter.

Accountability

Democratic accountability within the NHS comes through the Secretary of State to Parliament. The public, as citizens, elect an MP as their representative to make decisions on their behalf. This means that in health policy the only representation for citizens is at national level, which is far removed from where the decisions that affect them are made.

When the NHS was established, health services from several different traditions were brought together. There were the voluntary hospitals, where patients were treated for free and consultants, though not paid, were able to use their position at the hospital to attract private patients. Poor patients were also admitted to hospitals run by local authorities, often inherited from the Poor Law Commission in 1929. General practitioners had been brought into an insurance-based panel system in 1911, which was taken over virtually unchanged by the NHS in 1948. Local authorities were responsible for public health, health education and community services until 1974.

The National Health Service was set up as a separate organization in 1948 directly responsible to the Secretary of State, based on voluntary hospitals, because of opposition from the medical profession who wanted to preserve the independent status of doctors. Aneurin Bevan would have preferred the new National Health Service to be run by local government, since their elected councillors would have given the NHS democratic accountability. Historically health was an important part of the expansion of local authorities in the nineteenth century, in particular in housing, sanitation, parks and recreation. The public health movement, which resulted in the Public Health Act 1848, was a response to the cholera epidemics and crises in health caused by industrialization and the growth of cities. Reformers, like Edwin Chadwick, took on powerful interests such as the Water Boards, in order to ensure the provision of clean water and a healthier environment. From 1855 all metropolitan authorities had to appoint a medical officer of health, who was required to write an annual report on the state of public health in the area.

The decision to set up a separate structure for the NHS in 1948, managed by appointed rather than elected boards or authorities, meant that the medical profession was freed from lay control for the first time and health services removed from democratic accountability (Coast and Donovan, 1996). In addition, responsibility for health care, social care, and public and environmental health was fragmented. Ever since there has been an increasing slide away from democratic control over health services and a reduction in local authority involvement in health. In 1948 local authorities lost control over hospitals. In the 1960s the medical officer of health lost responsibility for welfare when social work became an independent profession. In 1974 community health services, including health education, were transferred to the NHS and the medical officer of health (whose name was changed to district community physician) became a part of the management team in the health authority. Public health inspectors became environmental health officers. However, local authorities have retained responsibility for many areas that affect health, the environment and the quality of life of local people. They are responsible for social services, housing, schools (where most health education takes place) and the environment (through planning, road safety, traffic management, street lighting, clean air, refuse disposal and recreation). They are also responsible for consumer protection which includes food safety and hygiene, weights and measures, food and drugs, as well as health and safety at work. The importance of local government in public health is increasingly recognized.

Accountability after 1990

Since 1990 it has been increasingly difficult for the public to become involved in planning and monitoring local health services. This may be partly because of the complexity of the new structures. Instead of one health authority responsible for all local health services, there were now many NHS trusts as well as private and voluntary sector providers and primary care commissioners. With the NHS and Community Care Act 1990, health authorities became responsible for purchasing – but not providing – health services, and their members (now called non-executive directors) were appointed by the Secretary of State for Health. At the same time local authorities became responsible for purchasing community care. There were suggestions from the government that health authorities, now freed from the responsibility for delivering services, could be 'champions of the people' (NHSME, 1992: 3). However, non-executive directors were not appointed for their knowledge of the local area or their links with the community but for their professional and managerial expertise. Few non-executive directors were women and very few were from minority communities (Cooper et al. 1995).

From 1990 hospitals and community services became separate self-governing NHS trusts, managed by a board made up of executive (salaried) directors and non-executive directors appointed by the Secretary of State. They were accountable to and monitored by the regional offices of the NHS Executive (NHSE). Surviving in the market meant that trusts had to compete with each other and with private providers for contracts and funds. Though it was useful to demonstrate that services were responsive to their users, the main responsibility of the board was to secure the market share – which might or might not benefit local people. Like the private sector they needed customers, but as long as the customers paid, it did not matter who they were.

The internal market introduced and justified more secrecy in trusts. Many NHS providers held board meetings in secret which they justified for commercial reasons since they were competing in a market with private providers who had no such constraints. Consequently, a Code of Openness was launched for the NHS in 1995, outlining the basic principles underlying public access to information about the NHS (NHSE, 1995). The NHS White Paper in 1997 stated that no information between NHS bodies could be kept in confidence for commercial reasons (Department of Health, 1997b).

No lines of accountability were identified for family practitioners when they became part of the NHS in 1948. Family practitioner services were administered by executive committees until 1974, when they were replaced by family practitioner committees who were charged with responsibility for managing services. These were in turn replaced in 1990 by family health service authorities who were amalgamated with health authorities in 1996. The division in the organization of primary and secondary care in the NHS was at last ended.

Because GPs are independent contractors, there has been little control over what they do, where and how they do it. This has resulted in enormous variations in the standards of service they provided. The Royal Commission on the NHS noted in 1979 that the poor quality of primary care in some inner city areas was one of the most significant problems facing the NHS. This was still true in the 1990s. In 1990 GP fundholding was introduced, whereby GPs, rather than the health authority, could purchase services directly for their patients. While health authorities facilitated and monitored fundholding, they had no powers to take action if fundholders failed to meet the standards set for them (Audit Commission, 1996).

In 1997 the White Paper, *A Modern and Dependable NHS*, put emphasis on accountability to local people. It gave health authorities stronger powers to improve the health of their residents through the development of health improvement plans, while primary care groups take over existing commissioning and fundholding arrangements. Primary care groups were required to have clear arrangements for public involvement, and were made accountable to health authorities through an annual agreement (Department of Health, 1997b). Arrangements were also proposed for clinical governance, whereby NHS trusts would have responsibility for quality standards in the same way as they had for finance (Department of Health, 1998a).

Community health councils

By the 1960s some of the problems caused by the lack of lay involvement and accountability in the NHS were recognized. Women's groups and self-help groups had shown how little notice health services took of their users and questioned the way health services were provided. Scandals in long stay hospitals for people with mental illness and mental handicap had shown what could happen when there was no public scrutiny and undermined public trust in professionals. As a consequence community health councils (CHCs) were introduced in the 1974 NHS reorganization as local watchdogs.

The initial proposal for CHCs came from the Conservative Government and was accepted, with some changes, by the incoming Labour Government. CHCs were set up as a committee of lay people to safeguard patients through more public involvement and scrutiny. Half the members came from local authorities, a third were elected by voluntary organizations and the remainder appointed by regional health authorities (which became regional offices of the NHS Executive in 1996). At the beginning most CHCs were set up with two staff and an office – sometimes in a high street or with a shop front and sometimes in hospital or health service property.

As statutory bodies, CHCs had some rights in relation to health authorities: to visit hospitals, to have access to information, to attend health authority meetings and to be consulted by NHS managers on changes in services. However, there was little guidance either for managers or CHCs on how these rights should operate and there were frequent disputes about their interpretation. In practice, if managers did not recognize CHCs' rights, they were unenforceable except by law. In some cases local authorities took legal action on behalf of CHCs against health authorities.

In 1974 CHCs were given the wide remit of 'representing the interests of the local community'. These terms of reference were interpreted very differently by different CHCs and the lack of guidance led to unacceptably wide variations between CHCs. A member of the public seeking information or assistance in making a complaint might get a very different service from one CHC than from another. In an attempt to clarify this, the Association of Community Health Councils for England and Wales identified five 'core' tasks (ACHCEW, 1991).

1 Acting as a voice for the local community.
2 Acting as a watchdog by monitoring local services.
3 Helping local people and local groups put forward their views to local NHS managers, in particular seeking out people whose views are not normally represented and acting as an advocate for them.
4 Providing information and advice to people who phone, write or come to the office.
5 Assisting people to make complaints.

No CHC can perform all these tasks to the same standard. Some CHCs have worked closely with community groups and involved local people in their activities, while in others members see themselves as a quasi-representative body. Some have focused on hospital visiting, assisting complainants or developing community initiatives. Some have worked closely and co-operated with NHS managers, while others have been in dispute with them. It is easy to look at an individual CHC and find it wanting in relation to a particular 'core' task. Where there are only two or three people employed, staff sickness, holidays, poor performance or personal conflicts can have a very disruptive effect on all its work. Research indicates that relationships between CHCs and the health service are most difficult in areas where CHCs have the fewest staff (Buckland et al., 1995). Many factors outside a CHC's control contribute to its 'effectiveness', such as the local financial situation in the NHS, and the attitude of NHS staff and their willingness to work with the CHC. The enormous variations in what CHCs do within limited resources make comparisons and evaluation very difficult (Hogg, 1996). The strengths and weaknesses of CHCs are summarized in Table 5.1.

In 1974 CHCs were an exciting new idea and there was still money around to develop new services. There were no precedents for CHCs to follow, examples for them to build on or expectations to fulfil. The freedom that they had in the way they worked led to innovation and CHCs made a significant impact in changing attitudes towards users in the NHS. Many activities now undertaken by the health service were pioneered by CHCs in the 1970s and 1980s: advocacy schemes, support for self-help groups and community networks, surveys of users' views,

Table 5.1 *Strengths and weaknesses of CHCs*

Factors affecting CHC performance	Strengths	Weakness
Lack of guidance and standards for CHCs	Flexible and responsive to local needs	No consistency in services provided by different CHCs
	Scope to develop new activities	Lack of focus in activities
		Limited monitoring or sanctions on a council of volunteers
Lack of enforceable rights for CHCs	'Managers can get on and manage'	'Watchdogs without teeth'
		Disputes with NHS about procedural rather than substantive issues
		Effectiveness may depend on co-operation of NHS management
Method of appointment of members	Members drawn from many different groups	Absentee members – and no sanctions
	Strong local authority links	Appointments of members on political affiliation
		No accountability
No line of accountability	Independent of NHS	No external audit or means of calling CHC to account
Resources	Resources not dependent on managers' perception of a 'good' CHC	Resources limited and do not reflect activities or quality of work

Source: Hogg (1996)

research on the unmet needs of disadvantaged groups, developing patients' charters, and providing information and advice.

CHCs were an example of back-of-the-envelope planning. They seemed a good idea in 1974, but what they would do, how they would work and how they would be accountable were never thought through. Since their heyday in the 1970s, there have been several attempts to get rid of them. In 1980 the government suggested that they were no longer necessary as the abolition of area health authorities meant that the smaller district health authorities could be in touch with the local community directly. With the introduction of general management in the mid-1980s, some felt that managers would be able to represent patients' interests and CHCs would no longer be needed. In 1990, with the split between purchasing and providing services, some felt health authorities could become the 'champions of the people', unfettered by the responsibility for directly providing services.

CHCs were created to operate in a very different world and their survival is remarkable in itself. However, the contradictions inherent in the way they were set up have become more evident. The situation reached a crisis for CHCs with the changes in the NHS and Community Care Act 1990. There was agreement that the functions provided by CHCs were important, that something must change, but not about how they should change. In 1996 the NHS Executive commissioned management consultants to review CHCs. Their report recognized the dilemmas of CHCs, with their limited resources, in attempting to offer information, advice and advocacy for patients and complainants, while at the same time contributing to planning and monitoring local services with limited resources (Insight, 1996). It suggested that CHCs should reduce their work with individuals, move out of high street, shop front premises and focus on planning. It did not, however, address the structural weakness of CHCs – how members are appointed, to whom they are accountable, and who should set standards and monitor CHCs. The conclusions were opposed by Conservative ministers even before the report was published. With the new complaints procedure introduced in 1996, which put emphasis on support for complainants, dropping this CHC function would have been ill-timed.

A different view of CHCs was taken by an 'expert' group commissioned by the NHS Executive, the Institute of Health Service Management and the NHS Confederation to make recommendations about public participation in the NHS. It suggested that CHCs should become 'professional scrutineers' with a remit to review the contribution of health and local authority services, audit policies of public authorities to assess their impact, and inspect health services and facilities. It suggested that CHCs could report to the Commission for Health Improvement, responsible for regulating standards in health service nationally (NHSE et al., 1998).

It is accepted that CHCs should be more focused in what they do, the question is which of the five functions identified by the ACHCEW could be dropped or taken on by others. Reluctant though many CHCs would be to lose direct contact with the public, independent information, advice and advocacy for individuals could be provided by other advice agencies, with resources and training. Monitoring or acting as 'scrutineers' was an important role of CHCs in 1974, when there were no other independent external mechanisms for audit and monitoring services. Now there are many other much better resourced agencies, including health authorities and primary care commissioners, the Audit Commission, the Social Services Inspectorate and now the Commission for Health Improvement. Users and their perspectives could be more routinely integrated into the work of all these bodies. The Social Services Inspectorate, for example, has recruited 'user consultants' as full members of their inspection teams visiting children's homes. User consultants are aged between 21 and 29 years and have themselves been in children's homes. They are trained to interview other children or to be 'inspectors' and are paid per session (Sone, 1993).

Some CHC functions cannot, however, be easily taken over by other agencies – in particular the role of encouraging and enabling smaller or disadvantaged groups or communities to have a voice in planning and running local services. This function must be independent and cannot be done by providers, health authorities or primary care groups. In developing this function, there is much that can be learnt from the experiences of CHCs in looking at possible future arrangements for enabling community participation. First, a community-based user body must be independent of the NHS and local authorities to have credibility with the public. CHC staff are employed by the NHS, and the regional offices of the NHS Executive are responsible for appointments, training and performance reviews of CHCs. If regional offices are responsible for setting standards and monitoring CHCs, there would be a clear conflict of interest. The Association of CHCs for England and Wales (ACHCEW) has argued that an independent body should be established to set standards and undertake training and development.

Secondly, accountability is important. CHC members are accountable to no one and are typical of people who join most committees – mainly white, middle class and middle aged. 'Typical' users do not join CHCs any more than they are elected to local councils or appointed to health authority or trust boards. This demonstrates the importance of developing new ways of enabling people to participate, in particular in linking with sections of the community who may not be able or wish to be involved in committees.

Thirdly, a new community-based user body needs to have a remit that reflects the concerns that people have around health, health care and social care rather than historical organizational divisions. It should have a wide remit with rights relating to hospitals, primary care, community care, and, possibly, other environmental and public services that affect health. Along with these rights there need to be responsibilities, and clear standards for the services that CHCs should provide and arrangements to monitor them.

Finally, a community-based body needs to be adequately resourced. Alhough money has been spent on health information services, patients' charters, surveys, citizens' juries and other methods of consulting users, these initiatives often sidelined CHCs and CHCs have remained as small isolated offices.

There has been an ambivalence and often hostility in government and managers' attitudes to CHCs, which illustrates the intrinsic difficulties of participation. Intellectually it is easy to appreciate the importance of participation and how this will lead to better decision making in the long term. In the short term, however, it is time-consuming, messy, challenging and can delay or destroy the best laid plans.

The voluntary sector

Voluntary organizations, through their members, generally have good information on the views of particular groups of users about what services are like and how they should be developed. However, giving their views to, and being consulted by, statutory bodies is not their main role. Some voluntary organizations were set up as philanthropic organizations, mainly before the establishment of the welfare state; many were set up by churches and religious organizations and the majority are still attached to them. Another tradition in the voluntary sector is that of self-help groups in which users and carers tend to take the lead. Voluntary organizations carry out many different activities that may include:

1 Providing services, such as helplines, rehabilitation or residential care for people with mental health problems, learning difficulties or drug or alcohol problems.
2 Acting as pressure groups.
3 Co-ordinating and providing resources to local groups, such as in local councils of voluntary service.
4 Self-help and mutual aid.
5 Fund raising – as medical charities and some hospital leagues of friends.

Most voluntary organizations do some or all of these activities, depending on their aims, the interests of their members and their funding. Often the lack of clarity about which function a group should pursue can lead to internal conflict and confusion (Handy, 1988).

In the past organizations in the voluntary sector often identified a need, and then approached health and local authorities for funding to provide a service to meet this need. Now the process is reversed. Local and health authorities will only fund services that fit within their priority areas and will not fund innovative or pioneering work which may incur extra costs and create new demands for services. As a result many voluntary organizations depend on service agreements or contracts. By working in this way, voluntary organizations may feel restricted in how far they can criticize the health or local authority on whom they depend for funding. Organizations need money to survive and funding through contracts is, in effect, a method of controlling their activities.

This brings a further problem. In order to compete with other providers, including private for-profit ones, voluntary organizations have to learn to speak the language of service agreements and contracts, and may become more hierarchical and professional. They may employ managers who have no personal experience of, or even particular commitment to, the health or personal problems that the organization aims to ameliorate. Thus managers may become distanced from the actual users, leading to conflict between the people for whom the organization was set up and the people who are considered to have the skills to manage it.

When looking for the elusive community 'voice', statutory services tend to look to the individuals and groups that they know and feel comfortable with. There is a danger that an 'elite' develops among the voluntary sector. The groups with contacts with statutory services may then be more likely to obtain funding and so their position becomes stronger in relation to other groups (Jewkes and Murcott, 1998). This may also further exclude those communities who are not well represented in the voluntary sector. Voluntary organizations that represent the interests of people from black or minority ethnic communities tend to be general and not specialist. As a result their voice is often not present in particular services, such as mental health services. This gap is serious since voluntary organizations are in a particularly good position to help people with mental health problems cope in the community and avoid the crises that mean they end up in hospital. Funding is needed to enable health service user groups that cater for black and minority ethnic communities to develop (Ahmed and Webb-Johnson, 1995).

Many user and self-help groups are informal, with little funding. They often start when a few people with a common problem come together as a mutual support group, people who are ill themselves or are dealing with other problems in their lives. They do not necessarily have the energy or skills to set up and maintain a group, let alone work with the health authority or local authority. Small groups, in particular, may need funds, practical help, training or emotional support to participate in consultations. Voluntary groups also need to feel that their contribution is valued, and the time and energy they put in is worthwhile. Participation is time-consuming and takes up resources and energy which would otherwise be directed elsewhere.

Consultation

Consultation was introduced formally to the NHS in 1974. In the 1970s and 1980s consultation acquired a specific meaning – referring to consultation that was a legal right of community health councils. Since 1974 health authorities have had to consult CHCs about any closure, substantial variation of use or development of services. In the event of a disagreement, CHCs had the right to appeal to the regional health authority and the Secretary of State.

These formal consultations generally involved hospital closures, and were the main power that CHCs had. They set a style for consultation in the NHS which antagonized managers and alienated the public. When the health authority was required to consult the public, it issued a document and circulated it to interested bodies to seek their comments. The information provided was often inadequate and written in ways that made it difficult to grasp the implications of the proposals. Consultation was often carried out when decisions had already been made: for example, even after services had 'temporarily' closed. Managers felt they needed to make quick decisions and resented the delays caused by consultation; the public felt that health authorities were merely going through the motions without wanting comments, making it all a waste of time.

Sir Roy Griffiths in his Management Inquiry in 1983 was not impressed with NHS consultation: 'by any business standards the process of consultation is so labyrinthine and the rights of veto so considerable, that the result in many cases is institutionalised stagnation' (DHSS, 1983: 12). Since the 1980s the nature of consultation and the areas for consultation have changed. The rights of CHCs to oppose closures and changes in services are less relevant, since many decisions are made by NHS providers who do not have to consult CHCs. Closures are often the result of earlier decisions made by health authorities about which services they are going to commission. In *Local Voices*, the NHS Management Executive recognized this: 'to give people an effective voice in the shaping of health services locally will call for a radically different approach from that employed in the past. In particular, there needs to be a move away from one-off consultation towards ongoing involvement of local people in purchasing activities' (NHSME, 1992: 1).

A further difficulty is the lack of a common language. A health authority asked local people what they thought common terms used in the NHS meant. Over half believed that secondary care meant 'less urgent NHS services', rather than simply hospital services. While over a third of respondents (36 per cent) thought that primary care was 'life saving services in the NHS' and a further 18 per cent thought it meant 'care delivered to children under eleven' (Spiers, 1998).

Public consultation has developed in two main directions since 1990: consultation based on localities and consultation on wider issues, such as rationing or choosing priorities for services, as outlined below.

Local areas

People are more likely to participate where they feel that discussions and plans are directly relevant to them and where participation is likely to have an impact. We tend to identify ourselves with the area where we live, shop and use services, which is a smaller area than that covered by local authorities or health authorities. Local or health authority areas cover many different communities, with differing and sometimes competing needs. For example, providing a health centre in one area may mean that a health centre will not be provided in a neighbouring area; a community hospital may be kept open in one town at the cost of one closing in another town.

In the 1970s and 1980s planning was generally undertaken on the basis of client groups, such as women, older people or people with mental health problems. In the 1980s, planning on the basis of localities instead of client groups was introduced in some rural areas in response to needs they perceived locally, drawing on experiences of community development projects working with disadvantaged communities (Balogh, 1996). In Exeter, health forums were set up by the CHC with funding from the health authority, to enable local people to contribute to planning. Locality planning or commissioning gained momentum in the 1990s when the introduction of GP fundholding meant that health authorities needed to find new ways of collaborating with GPs. In addition, mergers meant that health authorities were responsible for larger areas and so were more distant from their public.

These trends continued with the development of primary care groups and primary care trusts, which are expected to have clear arrangements for public involvement (Department of Health, 1997b). However, developing community links is relatively new in primary care. The Audit Commission (1996) found that users had little involvement in decisions about commissioning services made by general practices. GPs are both the providers and purchasers of services and there may be a conflict of interest in doing what is best for their individual patients and using resources in a cost-effective way.

The first patient participation group was set up in a GP practice in Wales in 1972 and since then groups have been set up in other practices. Patient participation groups involve patients and keep them informed about practice policies and decisions. Their activities vary widely and include commenting on services, co-ordinating volunteers, developing health promotion programmes and fund-raising. Volunteer schemes run by patient groups include lay visiting schemes for elderly housebound people, providing transport to the surgery, interpreting and collecting prescriptions (Pritchard, 1993). However, the inherent weakness of patient participation groups is that they tend to rely on the continued commitment of the GPs, so practices in urban areas with a transient patient population and smaller practices may not have the time or resources to nurture them. People who participate are more likely to be older women in higher socio-economic classes and, at the worst, this may lead to policies that perpetuate inequalities in access to services between practice patients (Agass et al., 1991). Some patients may, for example, prefer not to share the waiting room with homeless people or people who misuse drugs.

With a long tradition of privacy and independence, GPs resist the intervention of outsiders into the private relationship with their patients. Many GPs feel that, because of the close contacts they have with their patients, they are the best advocates for them. Community health councils have no legal right to be involved in services provided by GP practices. They cannot require information, insist on visiting premises or on being consulted. So far relationships between GPs and CHCs are not well developed (Joule, 1997).

There have been many different approaches to developing locality commissioning. In Newcastle localities were based on clusters of GP practices. In the most deprived of the localities, a researcher was appointed in 1994 to carry out a rapid appraisal (Freake et al., 1997). The results were presented at a conference attended by local people, health professionals and managers. There was agreement that the three priority areas for work were: supporting vulnerable families, young people, and those with mental health difficulties. A full-time community development worker, who was managed by the community health council, was appointed to facilitate participation. The participation of community groups led to a number of developments. These included a new service to meet the needs of vulnerable families by training five local people to provide them with peer support. Collaborating with local people meant that progress was slow but, in the end, the project had support and ownership from those living and working in the area.

Many health and social services overlap, and both health authorities and local authorities make assessments of the needs of their communities. In many areas health and local authorities have produced joint community care plans and children's services plans. This avoids duplication but is also important so that people feel that the issues they raise – whether about health or social care – are being addressed. Furthermore, local authorities have had more experience of consultation and participation than health authorities. In Islington, in North London, neighbourhood forums have been set up which hold open meetings where members of the public can discuss local services and develop local service agreements. Refuse collection was the first service discussed. The public were asked for their views about problems with services and there was a dialogue about the difficulties in implementing any suggestions. As a result, an agreement was negotiated with the neighbourhood forum about the service to be provided. The agreement was then publicized, along with a procedure for complaining if the terms were breached (Thomson, 1992). Everyone uses the refuse collection service, while other services, such as swimming pools and community care, are only used by a few people. For these services the process of negotiation needed to involve users and not just the neighbourhood forums. This approach could be useful in developing a local service, such as a health clinic or the appointment of a new doctor to a practice, where the ethnicity, gender or skills of the new partner may be important.

Choosing priorities

In the 1970s and 1980s, managers, the public, CHCs and unions were often embroiled in disputes about ward and hospital closures. These closures were sometimes made as part of the health authority's strategy to free funds to develop better services for elderly people, and for those with learning difficulties and mental health problems. These disputes led to calls for additional funding for the NHS but were not seen as 'rationing'. In the 1990s health authorities attempted to come to grips with the cash shortage by making explicit decisions about which services and what level of services they could afford to commission from their budgets. This raised the question of what legitimacy health authorities had to make these decisions, since they were not accountable to local people.

In the 1990s health authorities became interested in different ways that they could share (and legitimize) difficult decisions about which services should be provided and who should have priority to receive them. A famous and innovative example of consultation was in Oregon, USA, where the state developed a system to identify what services should be provided under Medicare, the publicly funded health service. A health services commission was created to develop a list of priority treatments through public involvement. A sample of local people were consulted about a list of diseases and interventions, and asked to rank how important they considered each to be. Then a line was drawn according to the funds available so that services and treatments above the line were funded and those below the line were not. Despite the many criticisms of the Oregon project, it was an ambitious attempt to unravel complex issues and provides some useful lessons (Kitzhaber, 1993).

First, it showed the importance of the quality of the information that is given to the public on which to base their judgements. The information may easily be biased by professionals who prefer to think positively about the benefits rather than the side effects of treatment. For example, in one survey based on the Oregon experiment (undertaken in City and Hackney in London), people were asked what services they thought were most important. Intensive care of premature babies was ranked number one, but when the wording was changed to intensive care of premature babies weighing less than one and a half pounds and not expected to survive, the ranking fell to ten (Blaxter, 1995).

Secondly, universal exclusions are not acceptable for most treatments, since there will generally be justifiable exceptions. Any exceptions need to be fair and decided on the basis of agreed clinical guidelines.

Thirdly, setting priorities needs to be based on how much the health of local people is likely to benefit ('health gain') and to take account of inequalities in the health status of different communities in the area. In the Oregon project, the interventions listed were not based on an assessment of needs, but on their specific effectiveness. For example, obesity – which is a major problem – was not included as there was limited evidence for the effectiveness of treatments (Honigsbaum et al., 1997). If decisions are based solely on the effectiveness of specific interventions, they will be unstable. People will appeal against the exclusion of treatments and individual decisions as new research is published and new evidence of effectiveness becomes available.

Fourthly, people tend to give priority to services that they use or can anticipate themselves or their family using. As a result some people's views will not be represented because they need a service which most people have no experience of or need for – such as for infertility or for learning difficulties. In Oregon, the choices reflected the fact that local people particularly valued a high quality of life and physical fitness. As a result disabilities fared badly and the US Congress rejected the consultations as they were felt to discriminate against people with disabilities and elderly people. Explicit rationing may be more 'democratic', but is likely to reflect public prejudices against some groups and may increase inequalities in access to health care.

Finally, different groups in the community have different priorities, and you still have to decide what weight to give to the claims of each group. In Oregon few people, in relation to the state population, were involved in making the assessment and so it did not necessarily mean the public accepted the decisions made by the health service commission. Some people may be unable or unwilling to put forward their views. Black people are often suspicious of services and distrust those in authority. They may have been dissatisfied or disillusioned by consultation exercises in the past and have experienced the ethnocentricity of health services, and white-dominated community health councils and voluntary groups. In Newham in London, where almost half the population is black, there is a Black and Ethnic Community Care Forum that has received joint financing from the health and local authority (Black and Ethnic Community Care Forum, 1992).

While there are difficulties in achieving a consensus in a society with many competing interests, there may be even greater problems in sticking to a policy. When faced with a real child who has a cancer that is probably untreatable, a rational decision by a health authority to cease treatment against the wishes of parents may seem inhumane. Public views in the abstract, and views about particular local services or services for ourselves and our families, may be quite different.

In order to have an informed debate about priorities, the public needs to know about cost-effectiveness and about the practical constraints on the decisions to be made. However, this information is complex and evidence may be contradictory and consequently difficult to present to the public. To overcome these difficulties the Institute for Public Policy Research and some health authorities have set up citizens' juries (Stewart et al., 1994). Citizens' juries are groups of between 12 and 25 citizens, selected to represent the general public, who get together to deliberate on a policy question. The jury generally sits for three to five days, hears evidence from expert witnesses and takes part in extended discussions before reaching a consensus. Though the commissioning authority does not have to abide by the decision, it must take account of it and give reasons for any disagreements. Citizens' juries have been used in Germany and the USA to help make decisions about road routes, rebuilding town centres and guidelines for welfare policies.

Citizens' juries are based on the belief that, given time and information, ordinary people can make complex decisions about issues that affect them – and that this is a better and more unbiased way of obtaining information than through pressure groups. In addition it also enables a more sophisticated analysis than is possible through questionnaires or surveys, which do not let people ask for more information and restrict the answers they can make. However, like any method of consultation, it depends on the goodwill of the body that is consulting. It decides how the jury is selected, what they will discuss and, largely, who will be called as expert witnesses. Most important, it decides whether to take any notice of the conclusions of the jury.

Underlying consultation exercises is the assumption that managers must manage and consultation should not interfere with their right to do so. Any consultation with the public is only advisory and managers can decide how far they want to listen to and take account of advice when they decide, for example, whether to commission new services for child and adolescent mental health or increase the number of hip replacements. As there is no democratic accountability, except at national level, the public has no right of reply.

Naomi Pfeffer (1995) forcefully expresses the exasperation of many involved in NHS consultation:

> In my neck of the woods, the general public have the temerity to defend hospitals threatened with closure, even though planners insist that we are 'over-bedded' . . . At CHC meetings, people talk about newsworthy health care issues, rather than debate strategies. Instead of discussing rationing, they insist on talking about cancelled operations, and how they cannot afford to buy treatments which are no longer provided by the 'new' NHS. . . . What the NHS needs is quasi-people, a new form of human species which unfortunately has not yet evolved. Quasi-people express themselves entirely in terms of patient satisfaction surveys; reproduce themselves in representative samples; make sensible comments on the latest ideas, such as a 'primary care-led NHS'; and even understand what it means to be a stake-holder in a healthy alliance; all this despite having no come-back where services are developed in a way which is inappropriate to their needs.

The 'representative' individual

Consultation exercises are often undertaken after decisions have been made and so it is important for user groups to put forward their views as early as possible. Many preliminary decisions are made in professional committees and sometimes lay or user members act as proxies for the wider community as members of these professional committees.

The concept of 'lay person' is frequently used as the public presence on professional committees, both at national and at local level, and the description is attached to people who are performing many different roles. As a term, 'lay' is defined negatively – simply the person is not a health service professional – rather than for any positive characteristics the person may have. A 'lay' representative can be a recent or present user, someone with links with the CHC or the voluntary sector, or a 'safe pair of hands' known to committee members. In a study of lay involvement, Brotchie and Wann found that there was enough consensus among 'lay' people to reach a definition: 'The lay person is someone who represents the public at large and whose starting point should be the user's or the patient's point of view' (1993: 5).

Lay people and users bring their own and other users' experiences to a committee and have a different perspective from professionals. Their value lies in the fact that they have different perspectives. Charlotte Williamson (1995) argues that there are three different categories of users: patients and carers, consumer groups, and consumerists. Patients and carers are not able to represent other patients' points of view because they seldom know what they are. Consumer groups, such as community, advocacy and self-help groups, are committed to identifying and articulating the interests of patients and other users. Consumerists are those users whose understanding of users' interests and concerns is wider and more abstract than that of any single user or patient group. Their perspectives are usually organized around general principles of equity and access, autonomy of and respect for the individual, support and advocacy, safety and redress as well as co-ordination and continuity of care.

The way that lay or user members are appointed and whom they 'represent' is determined by how much control the appointing body retains. Some managers have preferred to see the patient or carer, who is currently using or recently has used services, as the legitimate representative of other users, rather than consumer groups or consumerists. This approach is illustrated in maternity service liaison committees which were set up in 1984 as a forum where providers and professionals in hospitals and the community could work together to plan and co-ordinate local maternity services. It was accepted that there should be members representing the mothers' views from the beginning and later it was recommended that a lay member should be the chair of the committee (NHSE, 1996c). Some committees have tried to recruit women who have recently had a baby as members. Their value is seen to be in contributing their recent experiences of the service, not necessarily their contacts with other users or their understanding of the complex politics of maternity care. However, a new mother is unlikely to be able to contribute a wider user perspective, have the time or energy to understand the complexity of health service planning decisions or the technical arguments about the evidence base for guidelines and policies. She is likely to be recruited through maternity staff and so be sympathetic to them. She may be inhibited from expressing views as she may not want to antagonize professionals if she is likely to have another baby at the same unit.

Mental health service users have additional problems. Users' views which do not support professional interests can be rejected as irrational. Patients and their relatives are sometimes assumed to have the same interests; thus, when convenient, staff can seek relatives' rather than patients' views. As Lindow (1991) observed: 'Staff members expect to be patiently tolerant of a shaking client at their committee meeting. But are surprised and sometimes feel threatened by someone who is briefed on the issues. They then suggest that this person is not a proper service user because he or she is too articulate'.

There are also difficulties in asking children and young people directly for their views. Sometimes they are included in conferences or on working groups, but this may mean that children and young people are merely asked to contribute to a process over which they have no control. They may be expected to talk solely about personal issues or put over a particular message, which may not be what they would want to say. In 1995 CHAR (the Campaign for the Single Homeless) wanted young people to make a presentation to an Inquiry into Youth Homeless that it was undertaking. About twenty young people were identified by agencies and agreed to spend two residential weekends together exploring how best to get their views and experiences across. They used role-play and video interviews with members of the public and young people, comparing the different views the public and the young people themselves had about homelessness (Allard, 1996).

By offering membership of committees to recent users, others from CHCs, voluntary organizations or self-help groups, can be sidelined as they are not truly 'representative'. Because of their involvement with the CHC or voluntary organizations, they may be seen as partisan and different from other users because they have become 'professionals' (that is 'consumerists') or because their experiences are in the past and so their views can be discounted when desired. The test of 'representativeness' tends to be used against lay members, but not other members of the same committee: the representativeness of the consultant obstetrician or community midwife is not questioned. Nevertheless, the value of what you say does not depend on how many people you represent. If a clinical practice is poor, it does not matter if this information comes from a single complaint or from a quantitative survey of hundreds of patients.

Users themselves may dismiss other people who have not been through their experiences as unable to represent their views: someone who is not disabled cannot represent the views of people with disabilities; someone who has not been through the mental health system cannot represent the views of survivors. That people should be able to represent themselves wherever possible is a fundamental principle for developing user involvement. However, if taken too far this approach may weaken the position of more vulnerable users who have difficulty in putting forward their case. Many gay men who are HIV positive are part of a supportive community and are willing to speak out. The situation is different for women and people from minority ethnic groups who are HIV positive. They are often isolated and may not be willing to be identified, particularly if they have children who will suffer if their status is known. There will still be a need for consumerists.

Whoever and however they are appointed, one issue applies to all user or lay members of professional committees: how can an isolated individual, or even two, make an effective contribution to an established committee of professionals who all know each other? Because they are not 'experts', their views are not given the same weight or respect as those of other members. Professional members start from a position of superior knowledge and perceive themselves as objective in comparison to 'lay' people, who may rely on their own and others' experiences.

Using individuals as representatives of other users can give the appearance of involving users, but the conditions of involvement mean that they are often frustrated and ineffective. Some committees insist on confidentiality about their discussions which can leave a user member isolated. Unlike other members of the committee, confidentiality means that they are not supposed to seek information or advice from colleagues outside the committee. Whoever represents users' views – whether or not they are a recent or current user – should have close links with users themselves and continually refer back to this reference group.

Research into needs

Some health authorities have favoured scientific research as complementary to and, sometimes, as a substitute for participation. A 'scientific' or research-based approach to assessing what users need or want has definite attractions. Everyone belongs to many different communities – where they live or work, religious or cultural groups, ethnic origin communities, and their interest groups. The communities to which people belong shift and overlap, sometimes with shared, sometimes with conflicting, interests. Whose views are most valid? Consultation and talking to representative groups may increase participation by those who want to participate or those who have particular issues they want to push, possibly at the expense of other less articulate groups. Research is a way of learning about different groups in a systematic way. Furthermore, it avoids the confrontation that participation often involves. Members of the public can be aggressive and angry, and do not necessarily understand or follow the rules that NHS managers and professionals are used to.

Health authorities are required to base their health improvement plans and commissioning strategies on the actual needs of the local community rather than traditional patterns of services. They have used a variety of techniques. Epidemiological surveys, using morbidity and accident statistics, can give a useful indication of health problems and patterns of disease, especially if they focus on small communities. However, epidemiologists tend to rely on information that is already available and which can be measured statistically. Epidemiological methods alone cannot explain or understand the many different causes of ill health or the effect the environment has on health.

To complement epidemiological approaches, health authorities have undertaken surveys to find out local peoples' views, building on the surveys carried out by CHCs in the 1970s. Opinion polls and population surveys have been carried out to establish people's values, priorities and the health problems they see themselves as having. Large-scale surveys generally provide predictable information and do not show up the differences between localities. In order to be used to measure any improvements in health, surveys need to cover a small and relatively homogeneous population. Nevertheless, some people's views will be excluded because they are unable or unwilling to take part and this may undermine the credibility of the findings (McIver, 1993b).

Satisfaction surveys carried out over the last three or four decades show that those people who tend to express satisfaction may sometimes do so because they feel grateful or because they feel too vulnerable to criticize staff on whom they depend (Blaxter, 1995). Surveys do not engage people or encourage them to participate. Questions are set by managers and indicate to patients and carers what they are allowed to talk about. This is why, for example, so many patient satisfaction surveys found that people were happy to talk about food but did not comment on the areas which one would have thought were more important – the care they received from doctors and nurses and the quality of treatment (Carr Hill, 1992). Taking surveys out of the hospital setting may mean that people feel able to talk more freely. When they feel able to talk more freely, they may tell a different story about their experiences. Satisfaction is also influenced by factors that superficial surveys do not uncover, such as people's previous experiences of health care, their reasons for seeking care, as well as their expectations and beliefs about what a health service should be like.

Qualitative methods give participants more opportunity to talk about their own concerns than quantitative methods. Participants can contribute on their own terms and identify issues that are important to them. For example, focus groups are a useful way of gathering information, bringing together individuals who have a particular condition or use a particular service. They are increasingly used in planning and commissioning services in order to obtain local views about health and health care. Critical incident techniques, on the other hand, use semi-structured interviews to ask respondents to recall the details of a particular experience or incident that they felt to be important (Fitzpatrick and Bolton, 1994). Finally, consumer audit is a qualitative approach to obtaining feedback developed by the College of Health, a national consumer organization. It provides a profile of patients' and carers' views of particular services, using a range of techniques such as surveys, observation, semi-structured interviews and focus groups (College of Health, 1994). Different ways of assessing needs and obtaining user views are summarized in Table 5.2.

In the 1980s there was a re-emergence of a public health movement in the UK. The Leeds Declaration, *New Ways to Understand and Solve Public Health Problems*, was drawn up at an international workshop held in 1993. It highlighted the importance of users in research and the validity of their views, and emphasized that qualitative research was needed to obtain a full picture. It also recognized that research itself will do nothing to change people's lives and that knowledge about the causes of ill health should be used to promote better health. Three years after the Declaration, changes had been slow. Public health and consultation had been taken up with issues around rationing and cost control rather than developing new ways of consulting local people (Long, 1997).

However, the principles in the Declaration are still relevant. Assessing the needs of particular communities has been successfully undertaken by directly involving local people. For example, local people themselves can

Table 5.2   *Ways of finding out about users*

Method	Advantages	Disadvantages
Epidemiology	Standardized to allow comparisons	Can lead to biomedical reductionism and not reflect total environment
		Limited to measurable and available data
		Often reflects provider, not user concerns
Questionnaires • self completion • structured	Simple to administer Standardized to allow comparisons	Often reflect provider, not user concerns Limit the user response
Qualitative methods • focus groups • observation • consumer audit • critical incident techniques	Allow users to choose areas to talk about Provide information on areas that need further investigation	Require skill and training of researchers May produce idiosyncratic results

be used as interviewers in order to obtain information from people who view outsiders with suspicion, such as travellers or residents of some housing estates. In one area HIV transmission and health awareness among 'new age' travellers were investigated by a team of new age travellers with support from voluntary sector workers and academics (Oliver and Buchanan, 1997).

Community-based needs assessment can run into difficulties if it does not involve local people appropriately (Edwards, 1996). First, the objectives of involving people in needs assessment are sometimes confused. Is the intention to educate the public, give the health authority legitimacy for its decisions, or make the case for more money for health care? Secondly, communities may not be aware of their 'needs' or may have low expectations. Surveys can achieve little without more basic community development work. Thirdly, sometimes the methods used in needs assessment are dubious. Needs assessment often relies on key informants who can act as proxies for their communities. This can lead to bias if health authorities rely on proxies, particularly as the authorities are in a position to select their own 'proxies'.

Edwards (1996) also found that community-based needs assessment often had little impact on actual purchasing decisions. There was no incentive for managers to take account of the findings of research unless it suited their purpose. In addition, they could suppress the findings. Therefore, it can be argued that community-based needs assessment is more appropriately undertaken by working closely with communities and contracting local voluntary groups and community health councils to undertake it.

Empowering communities

Some public health professionals have focused on research and epidemiology, while others have looked at ways of 'empowering' local people. In the 1970s and 1980s some health promotion professionals began to work with disadvantaged communities to help them improve their health, moving away from the top-down approach of the older tradition of public health. The healthy living centres initiative launched by the Labour Government in 1997 recognized the value of working with disadvantaged communities, on their own terms, in promoting health (Department of Health, 1998c).

Healthy living centres, however, are not new. The first community health project was developed in Peckham in the 1930s. The Peckham Health Centre was a pioneering experiment, set up by doctors disillusioned with the traditional medical approach (Scott-Samuel, 1990). It was a centre which provided a combination of leisure, nutrition, health and education. Local families joined up and participated in the development and the running of the centre – the only requirement was a medical examination so that the impact of the centre on the community might be assessed. The centre started with healthy people and worked to create circumstances in which people were able to cultivate their physical, mental and emotional health. It was closed in 1950, after operating for only eight years divided by the Second World War. It closed partly because of financial problems, partly due to government indifference and, perhaps, because it was expected that the new National Health Service would make it redundant.

These experiences were forgotten. Community health initiatives and the 'new public health' developed from the women's movement, civil rights movement in the USA and self-help movements that emphasized the importance of speaking for oneself and valued experience over professional knowledge. It recognized the limits of much of modern health care and the inequity in access to health care. Community development approaches also had international roots in the World Health Organization's 'Health For All' (Chapter 7).

The first neighbourhood health projects in the UK were set up outside the NHS in the 1970s. They were very varied, but there were common themes, in particular they saw health in social rather than medical terms and took a collective rather than an individual approach to solving community problems. Activities depended on what local people felt was important and might include a mother and toddler group, a support group for people dependent on tranquillizers, schemes to cope with drug dealing in the area, or campaigns to get house repairs done or cars excluded from the streets where children play. A review in 1996 commissioned by the Department of Health to look at 'community well-being centres' and co-operatives found over three hundred projects (Gaskin and Vincent, 1996). Although there were wide variations in the scope and scale of the projects, there were some common features. Participation and ownership by local people was central, although the extent varied. Some were 'top-down', initiated by health or local authorities, while others were initiated by voluntary organizations or the communities themselves. These centres now provide the basis for the development of healthy living centres. Times have changed since the 1950s when the Peckham Centre closed. Near the site of the original centre, the Canal Head Health and Leisure Centre has been built, funded by the health authority and Southwark Council.

One longer-term initiative is the 'Healthy Cities' project, an international network of collaborating cities initiated by the World Health Organization as part of its Health For All strategy. A key part of the definition and objectives of a 'Healthy City' is the involvement of citizens in creating conditions for the promotion of health and well-being. Glasgow, which has one of the poorest health records in the UK, is a 'healthy city'. As a healthy city, all the activities that take place in the city are recognized to have some impact on the health and well-being of local people and all agencies are involved in developing a broad-based City Health Plan

(Black, 1996). The European Network of Health Promoting Schools is a research and development initiative by the World Health Organization and the European Commission. In England the Health Education Authority worked with 38 schools to demonstrate how schools can promote health in their style of teaching, learning, relationships, and eating habits (Hamilton, 1997).

Another international initiative that works with local communities is Agenda 21. In 1992 the 'Earth Summit' in Rio de Janeiro, set out in Agenda 21 the actions that needed to be taken at international, national and local level to promote a healthy environment. The approach is based on grass-roots voluntary action in partnership with local authorities and business. In London, the Association of London Government set up a health task group that identified key priorities including better housing, reduction in crime, better air quality and better opportunities for children, as well as the designation of London as a 'healthy city' under the WHO programme.

However, there are criticisms of the new public health. Community development approaches do not give quick results and require long-term investment. Unfortunately the funding provided for 'innovative' schemes is generally short term and not part of a general strategy or mainstream funding. Healthy living centres, for example, are to be funded from the National Lottery. In addition, community development approaches are difficult to evaluate because they are mainly about increasing people's self-confidence and developing better relationships between professionals and community members. Gaskin and Vincent (1996) found that monitoring and evaluation were often inadequate because insufficient funds were available for this.

Petersen and Lupton (1996) argue that the new public health is still based within the framework of the health service and local government. The public health agenda is set by professional experts and is closely aligned with official objectives. Professionals may be concerned with physical health, such as infant mortality, immunization or heart disease, whereas people themselves may give priority to stress, housing or community safety. However well meaning they are, professionals may not always understand how alienating their scientific knowledge and assumptions are for disadvantaged people.

Community development should enable people to solve problems and meet their needs as they see them. Unlike traditional health education, community development approaches do not expect individuals to help themselves (and blame them if they fail), but they do expect communities to improve their environment and health. There are limits to what can be achieved by communities; poverty, unemployment, crime, poor housing and environmental pollution are determined by political decisions at national and international level. Actions at local level by local authorities, health authorities and community groups are likely to be marginal without national direction, backed up with resources.

Conclusions

There is sometimes confusion about the purpose of 'participation'. Does it mean the same as 'involvement'? Is it to educate citizens or to enable them to take part in decisions? Is it to 'legitimate' and validate the decisions that purchasers and providers of services make on behalf of the public? Is the purpose to improve democratic accountability? There is an increasing amount of consultative activity in the NHS; but this is mainly to an agenda set by managers, on terms that they decide, and does not involve sharing decisions or power.

Managers do not often address the question of why people should bother to participate and what benefits they can expect from participating. We may exert our right as citizens to give our views or not as we wish, and vary in our motivation and ability to do so. It is hard to participate if you are homeless, work long hours, have young children, are illiterate, have communication or access difficulties, or are from a minority ethnic group. Other things are more pressing. You may also be reluctant to spend time 'participating' if you feel services are being properly provided, do not affect you or that nothing will change as a result. All these are good reasons to decide not to spend leisure time on 'participation'.

The approaches described in this chapter are summarized in Figure 5.1. Underlying each approach are beliefs about public participation, the nature of the contribution that users can make and how far managers do or should maintain control over the terms of the participation. All these approaches have a place in increasing public and community involvement in health.

Local arrangements for community participation must be flexible and concentrate on ensuring that there are opportunities for people to participate, should they wish to. This involves attention to details – such as access and timing of meetings, training and support. Managers must be honest about whether the consultation is to give information (since they do not see an alternative to their proposals) or genuinely to listen to local people and take their views into account. It is important that those concerned are clear why a particular approach or technique is appropriate and how they will follow up any consultation. In addition, there will need to be independent arrangements for enabling smaller and less organized voices to be heard. Community health councils could provide the basis for an independent framework for dialogue that enables disparate and conflicting views to be heard. This would require changes in their role, the way members are appointed and their accountability.

Without also addressing accountability and democracy, it may be difficult to make 'participation' attractive for people. People will not participate unless they are convinced that it will result in change and is related to decision making. In the UK people are familiar with what participation means, but local decision making is limited by the restrictions placed on the activities of local and health authorities by central government.

	Values and assumptions	Aims	Comments
Democratic accountability	People who make decisions on behalf of others should be accountable for them, requiring open decision making	To call to account	No democratic accountability at local level
Research	Research methods are more objective and can identify needs and obtain feedback from local people	To find the facts to inform management	Local people as source of information
Consultation exercises	Managers need to manage but also take account of local people's views	To validate and/or legitimize decision making	Local people as advisers, without sharing decisions
Community health councils	Local people need a channel to keep them informed and help them express their views to the NHS	To enable the views of different sections of the community to be heard	Too much variation in effectiveness and lack of accountability
User groups and voluntary organizations	Voluntary organizations have knowledge and experience of services and can contribute to planning and management	To put forward the views of particular users or communities	Focuses on specific services and interests
Empowering communities	Local people, particularly from disadvantaged communities, need assistance to articulate their needs and act to achieve them	To 'empower' disadvantaged communities to influence local services and their environment	Requires long-term investment

Figure 5.1 *Approaches to community involvement*

This has undermined the legitimacy and status of local authorities in the eyes of the public. In the nineteenth century, local authorities gained new power and legitimacy from their role in public health; their decline may be a consequence of their loss of this role to the NHS. In contrast, in France there is more enthusiasm for participation because people have confidence in the autonomy that municipalities have to make decisions (Council of Europe, 1994). In Spain people are less familiar with 'participation' and have had little experience of it – following a forty-year dictatorship under Franco. However, more decisions are made locally and this allows greater scope for enabling people to participate. With changes in the organization of the NHS and local authorities, there is increased interest in the proposal that local authorities should become the commissioners of health and social care (Hunter, 1995). This would bring together again responsibility for public health (now with the health service) and the management of public health (now with local authorities), and introduce again democratic accountability with services.

6

CITIZENS

Every government carries a health warning.

Badge slogan, 1976

Richard Tawney wrote in 1931:

> Health is a purchasable commodity of which a community can possess, within limits, as much or as little as it cares to pay for. It can turn its resources in one direction and 50 000 of its members will live who would otherwise have died; it can turn them in another and 50 000 will die who would otherwise have lived.

Public policies have an enormous impact on health by putting resources where they are most likely to improve health – income, environment, food safety, clean water and good housing – or not. However, taking action is not quite so simple. There is an enormous distance between people's everyday experiences and national policy making and it is hard for the public – as users and as citizens – to participate in national debates about health and health services. There is no overall national health policy, and the processes of government and policy making are complex and often obscure. Commercial, professional and user organizations all attempt to influence policies in their own favour. However, in comparison to professional and commercial lobbies, the user movement is unorganized, under-resourced and disparate.

In this chapter we consider how the public – as citizens and users – influence national policies and what the barriers to wider participation are.

Ministers and Parliament

National policies are made by ministers who are accountable to Parliament. Electors are represented by MPs, who are voted in or out every five years or so, but there is usually little opportunity to use a vote to influence health policy. People can lobby their MP, who can ask questions in Parliament, put forward a private member's bill and move for an adjournment debate. Members of Parliament sit on select committees, which can question civil servants and ministers about government policies. The public and user organizations are able to give evidence to select committees and this can be an important way of getting views heard.

Members of Parliament are concerned with representing their voters – but on many issues there will be little consensus. Some local people will want more public funding for health care, while others will want less. Some will feel passionately about women's right to have an abortion, while others will feel just as passionately about the rights of the unborn child. For any pressure group, it is important to identify champions in Parliament who will keep raising the profile of the cause.

The theory is that ministers decide policy and civil servants carry it out. Though ministers are far too busy and overworked to maintain a firm hand on what goes on in their departments, ministerial accountability means that politicians and the civil servants who work for them are deemed to be democratically accountable. As a consequence, they may not feel the need for transparency or public participation in order to legitimate or validate their actions and policies. The role of central government was strengthened in 1996 when regional offices of the NHS Executive replaced regional health authorities.

Ministers also have great powers of patronage. In September 1995 ministers made 3889 appointments to NHS bodies. Patronage in appointments to NHS trust boards was important during the implementation of the NHS internal market in the early 1990s, where non-executive members who supported the reforms could be relied on not to criticize government policies openly. Similar criticisms were levelled against the Labour Government as they made their first appointments to NHS bodies in 1997. Concern about how public appointments were made led to the appointment of a Commissioner for Public Appointments in 1995, following the *Nolan Report* on standards in public life (House of Commons Public Service Committee, 1996).

Government departments and national strategies

Policy is not made by a single decision but is often the result of an accumulation of decisions. In fact, much political activity is about avoiding decisions and maintaining the status quo. This is particularly true of health policy, where several government departments with different objectives make policies that affect health and which may work against each other. The competition and lack of co-ordination between government departments hampers public involvement. Successful lobbying requires accurate targeting of the right person, at the right level in the organization, at the right time. It is difficult to influence decisions if you do not know where decisions are being made, when, and by whom.

Conflicting interests

There is no national health strategy covering all government departments and so confusions and contradictions abound. Government departments may make decisions that affect health but may have objectives that are contrary to those of the Department of Health. Each department has close links with organizations representing the particular interests whose co-operation it needs to achieve its objectives. The Department of Health, for example, needs to work with the British Medical Association and, to a lesser extent, other professional and staff groups. It also needs to work with pharmaceutical companies in order to ensure the safe and effective use of medicines, while at the same time promoting the medical equipment and pharmaceutical industries. These aims may be in conflict and the National Consumer Council has recommended that the Department of Health's sponsorship of the pharmaceutical and medical industries should be transferred to the Department of Trade and Industry. The DTI is responsible for promoting trade and exports – including those of the pharmaceutical and medical equipment industries, as well as industries that directly damage health like tobacco and alcohol. Similarly, the Ministry of Agriculture, Fisheries and Food (MAFF) is responsible for both protecting consumers and promoting agriculture and fisheries. The protection of consumers requires that MAFF should act as soon as it is known that there is the possibility of harm, while the protection of producers and the economy require MAFF to make absolutely sure about the scientific evidence before acting – even though this can take years to obtain.

As an example, each department has its own policy on tobacco. Policies that reduce smoking and alcohol use will affect jobs and exports. The Treasury collects the taxes, the DTI and the Department of Employment are concerned to maintain jobs. Sport and the arts have benefited from sponsorship by tobacco companies. Thus health is not necessarily a major consideration as these departments formulate policy.

Co-operation between government departments

Co-operation between government departments is essential for a health strategy that promotes health and is not just concerned with providing health care. However, problems in developing comprehensive national health strategies are not new. *The Beveridge Report* of 1942 identified the five giants to be defeated: want, disease, ignorance, squalor and idleness. Beveridge designed a comprehensive welfare system based on a free national health service, child allowances and full employment. However, these goals have never been fully realized.

Attempts to develop overall government health strategies have been frustrated by the strength of individual departments. In the mid-1970s there was a failed attempt to improve co-ordination between government departments: the joint approach to social policy (known as JASP). The

Social Exclusion Unit – a ten-year initiative to tackle inequalities – set up in the Cabinet Office in 1997, bears a resemblance to JASP. It was set up because the problems of social exclusion, such as failure at school, unemployment and crime, are woven together and solutions need co-ordination and co-operation across government departments. The reasons for failure, David Hunter (1997) argues, are still relevant. The joint approach of JASP failed because most ministers were more interested in quick results and did not understand its relevance for the long term.

Many government departments are involved directly in tackling inequalities in health: Social Security, Environment, Education and Employment as well as Health. However good the evidence for the importance of housing, income and employment for improving the health of the nation may be, accepting inequalities as important determinants of health has enormous financial and political implications. The reluctance to accept the political implications of inequalities can be seen in the reaction to *The Black Report* in 1980. The Research Working Group on Inequalities in Health was convened by the then Labour Government, under the chairmanship of Sir Douglas Black, President of the Royal College of Physicians. By the time the Group reported, however, there was a Conservative government. The report recommended government intervention to tackle child poverty, the provision of free school milk and free school meals, more spending on housing, investment in day care, antenatal facilities, and home helps and nursing services for disabled people. It was published in 1980 on August Bank Holiday Monday in the hope of avoiding publicity; the government did not like the report's findings. They preferred to see citizens as responsible for their own health and believed that economic prosperity would generate personal wealth and, by 'trickling down', benefit everyone in society (Townsend and Davidson, 1988). The recommendations of the *Black Report* were ignored and inequalities in health increased during the 1980s and 1990s. In 1997 the Labour Government, in addition to setting up the Social Exclusion Unit, appointed the first Minister for Public Health and, building on the previous Health of the Nation initiative, launched a public health strategy – *Our Healthier Nation* – to tackle the root causes of ill health and, in particular, inequalities (Department of Health, 1998b). However, critics felt that the omission of targets to reduce inequalities weakened the thrust of this strategy.

The importance of co-operation between government departments can be illustrated in the ways the government promotes the health of children and young people. The Department of Education and Employment is responsible for health promotion for school children and nutritional standards in school meals. Since the Second World War free school milk and meals were seen as important in promoting health in adult life and were identified in the *Black Report* as important in reducing inequalities in health. However, in 1980 school meals were deregulated, leaving it to local education authorities to decide policy. In many areas school meals were replaced by sandwiches and most school meals staff were dismissed. In schools run by the Inner London Education Authority (ILEA) the school meals service was actually providing less than a quarter of the 1978 recommended daily allowance for nutrients when it was abolished in 1990 (Jenkins, 1991). The Social Security Act 1986 made it illegal to provide free milk and free school meals to any pupil unless their parents were receiving Income Support. The government Committee on the Medical Aspects of Food Policy (COMA) carried out a survey in 1983 to look at the consequences of the deregulation of school meals. It concluded that the main sources of energy in the diets of British school children were bread, chips, milk, biscuits, meat products, cake and puddings. School meals and tuck shops were a major source of these foods (COMA, 1989). Its findings were an official secret until they were eventually published in 1989.

Lobbying government

In formulating policy, government departments take advice from advisory committees, regulatory bodies and key professional, commercial and voluntary organizations. They produce consultative documents: Green Papers are primarily for discussion, while White Papers outline proposed legislation. Government departments seek comments on these from a wide range of organizations. However, as with local consultations, by the time the consultative document is published, deals have often already been made behind the scenes.

Decisions about health policy are made following lobbying, both in public and private, by interest groups who use the best methods available to them to get attention for their causes and to influence policy. There are many pressure groups with an interest in health, representing professional, commercial and public interests. There are often shared interests between these groups and alliances form from time to time between them. Pressure groups vary in power and in the extent to which they have access to people who make decisions. The government needs the support of some groups in order to make policies workable and they often have a close relationship with government and share power. The government does not need the co-operation of user or public interest groups, and they are easy to ignore as they are fragmented and do not work as a co-ordinated lobby. Sometimes they are dominated by professional or commercial interests.

Lobbying does not stop when policy is made. Policy decisions by government do not necessarily lead to changes in local services, especially where resources are not there to implement them. Consequently, many well-intentioned national policies fail: for example, in the 1970s priority was given to improving the 'Cinderella' services (including services for older people and people with mental illness, learning difficulties or disabilities). In spite of this there were few improvements in these services.

In the 1990s, while the government pushed ahead with the primary care-led NHS, health authorities were proposing to close community hospitals to meet their financial targets. Much of the work of voluntary organizations is not so much trying to influence national policy as trying to persuade managers to implement national policies in local services.

Advisory committees

The government takes advice from advisory committees of experts. Public interest organizations may be invited to nominate a member to some committees, in particular where their remit involves operational issues such as standards for services, though their nominees may be vetoed. Often lay members are drawn from an establishment list of the 'great and the good' and come from a similar background to other members. They may not challenge professional or other interests or have a support or reference group to ensure that they are representing more than their own personal views. Statutory regulatory bodies, such as the General Medical Council and the General Dental Council, have lay members appointed by the Privy Council, who are mainly other health professionals with no background in users' concerns.

MAFF increased consumer representation in the 1980s and 1990s in a more systematic way than other government departments. MAFF set up a Food Advisory Committee in 1983 to advise ministers on changes to labelling, permitted additives and novel foods which has two consumer members. In the wake of food scares, a consumer panel was set up in 1989 which was made up of individuals nominated by consumer groups. The panel had some success, though there were issues about how MAFF defined 'consumers'. Staff and chairs of consumer organizations and single issue groups such as the Coronary Prevention Group, Action for Information on Sugars, and Parents for Safe Food were excluded as consumer representatives. The National Consumer Council (1994a) pointed out that it is naive to think that ordinary consumers would have the confidence, and some of the skills and knowledge required to contribute to the panel. The Labour Government soon after their election in 1997 announced that a Food Standards Agency would be set up to protect public health in relation to food, which would have a majority of members with a public interest background (MAFF, 1997).

How 'experts' are defined and chosen for advisory committees determines the subsequent advice it gives. For example, the Calman/Hine Committee looked at cancer services, but had no user or lay member (Department of Health, 1995). Though the *Calman/Hine Report* noted that psychosocial care was important to patients and carers, it did not consider how it might be provided or mention it in the summary of recommendations. In contrast, the expert committee on maternity services was different. Of the nine members, there was a GP, a consultant obstetrician, a paediatrician, a public health professional and a professor of midwifery.

The remainder were 'lay' people. The chair and seven out of the nine members were women. As a result the report, *Changing Childbirth*, largely reflected what user groups had been campaigning for (Department of Health, 1993). The choice of 'experts' was important in this. A group dominated by obstetricians would have come out with different recommendations.

The way an issue is defined determines the choice of 'experts' and influences subsequent government actions. This can be illustrated in the way that the government handled the BSE crisis. Bovine Spongiform Encephalitis (BSE) was first identified in cattle in 1986 by the government's veterinary service and was reported to the public in June 1987. As it was seen only as a problem for farmers, the Department of Health were not informed until March 1988 – almost a year and a half after it was first identified. The government set up two scientific advisory committees and followed their advice. The problem lay in the choice of members for the committees who were not epidemiologists but scientists from orthodox backgrounds, who saw BSE as an animal not a human problem (Maxwell, 1997). They were not looking at the public health implications of the risk for humans of contracting Creutzfeldt-Jakob Disease (CJD) from eating beef. However, the commercial and farming lobbies, who had so much to lose by stronger regulations, must have had some influence, since British bovine materials were banned from use in medicinal products in 1989, but the risks from food were not acknowledged publicly until 1996. The way the crisis was handled caused serious long-term problems for the country, its relationships within Europe, and an as yet unknown number of people who will contract CJD.

Users and 'lay' people are often excluded from committees defined as 'technical', though their deliberations have enormous implications for the public. The Committee on the Safety of Medicines was set up by the Medicines Act 1968 to advise the Department of Health. This followed concern that the pharmaceutical industry was out of control and the market was being flooded with undesirable drugs. The Thalidomide tragedy in the 1960s, when women gave birth to babies with limb deformities after taking the drug for nausea during pregnancy, led to calls for greater regulation. In 1989 the Medicines Control Agency was set up to take over the work of the old licensing division of the Department of Health. The pharmaceutical industry funds the Medicines Control Agency and the Committee on Safety of Medicines through licence fees. Until recently it charged £250 admission to its annual meeting, ensuring that the overwhelming attendance was from company representatives (Medewar, 1992).

The Committee on Safety of Medicines is now an expert committee of the Medicines Control Agency and advises it on the licensing of medicines and on urgent safety matters which require further investigation. It also promotes the collection and investigation of reports of adverse reactions to medicines. The Committee has been criticized by consumer groups for relying on doctors and drug companies for its information, and for not exerting any real control over the way drugs are used and marketed. Professional members may have close connections with pharmaceutical companies – and it may be difficult to find experts without these links. The National Consumer Council pointed out that there were questions about the appointment of experts 'since there can be few eminent or appropriately qualified individuals who are not in some way beholden to the industry' (NCC, 1991: 86). There are no consumer or user representatives on the Committee on the Safety of Medicines.

Before the 1997 general election the pharmaceutical industry published a manifesto: *What Industry Needs from Government*. In response, the Insulin Dependent Diabetes Trust (IDDT) produced their 'patients' manifesto' *What Patients Need from the Pharmaceutical Industry and Government*. This suggested that a strategy group working across government departments be set up to review pharmaceutical issues. This group would include patients (not professional representatives of patient groups), and representatives of the Departments of Health, Trade and Industry, the Treasury and the Office of Fair Trading. Patients would be involved in panels that monitor and license drugs; also, patients, carers and pharmacists would be able to make direct reports of adverse drug reactions (IDDT, 1997b).

Openness and access to information

A further problem for lobby groups has been the long-established culture of secrecy in British government. Openness and public scrutiny is particularly vital because of the potential conflict of interest within government departments, and their close links with commercial and professional interests. It is important for consumers to see how decisions are made and whether commercial or other interests have dominated decisions There have been major shifts since the days of the Official Secrets Act 1911, which was finally replaced in 1989. Section 2 of this Act decreed it illegal for an employee of the government to disclose any official information and for anyone else to receive it. Furthermore, the public interest defence was excluded. Secrecy benefits pressure groups who prefer to operate behind the scenes.

The Code of Practice on Access to Information in Government came into force in April 1994, following concern about standards in public life. The Code was not enforceable and did not offer access to actual documents, only information from those documents. Information could be withheld to protect commercial confidentiality, which even included the cost of printing the Citizen's Charter, the price at which hospitals were sold off by health authorities and the cost to the NHS of prescriptions for emergency contraception (Frankel, 1994). The Code fell far short of a freedom of information act such as exists in the USA, Canada, Australia, New Zealand, France, Sweden, Denmark, Norway, Greece and the Netherlands. In 1997 a White Paper was published proposing a freedom of information act (Cabinet Office, 1997). This is of great importance in enabling the public and user groups to scrutinize the way decisions are made and identify the lobbies that influence decisions. Any radical measures probably need to be introduced as soon as a new government gets into office. Once established in power, government departments have their own secrets and a vested interest in restricting access to information.

Secrecy has been particularly great in the licensing and regulation of medicines. The deliberations of the Medicines Control Agency are secret under Section 118 of the Medicines Act 1968 and no government minister or official can publish any information about a drug company or its research connected with the licensing of medicines. Breaches of the law carry a maximum sentence of two years' imprisonment. Section 118 was originally designed to protect commercial secrets but is used as a blanket ban on all information, including information about adverse reactions, deaths caused by a drug, and the types of drugs used by the NHS and their cost to the tax payer.

The exclusion of consumers makes it hard, if not impossible, for people to be informed, responsible about taking medicines or to participate in their own health care. Consumers need access to the studies on which decisions are based as well as the reasons for these decisions. In the USA the Food and Drugs Administration prepares a summary of its decisions which is available through the Internet. Reports of its inspections of British pharmaceutical companies are available to the public from the FDA who visit UK firms which export to the USA. In contrast, in the UK, reports of inspections undertaken by the Medicines Control Agency are restricted. A private member's bill attempted to repeal Section 118 of the Medicines Act in 1993, with the support of the British Medical Association and consumer groups. This was blocked by some MPs who declared their interests as advisers to pharmaceutical companies. The Association of the British Pharmaceutical Industry threatened that, if the bill became law, member companies would boycott the British drug licensing system. Not all countries are so secret. The Swedish Medical Products Agency publishes a regular newsletter with comparative information about the drugs it approves which is available to the public. The pharmaceutical industry opposed this extension of information about drugs in 1985, arguing that it would have a disastrous effect on the Swedish pharmaceutical industry. However, it did not cause the problems that the industry predicted.

Missing debates

There are also incentives for politicians to evade open debates on sensitive issues in order to avoid the criticism that goes with controversy. Some major policies are introduced without an explicit decision and so are implemented before the public or voluntary sector have a chance to give their views and point out what changes would mean. An example of this is the withdrawal of the NHS from continuing care in the 1990s. Though it has never been clear whether the NHS or local authorities were responsible for the continuing care of elderly people, in general older people who needed medical or nursing care were in NHS hospitals, while local authorities looked after the others. The big difference was that NHS care was, and is, free, while local authority care is means-tested. Between 1990 and 1994 many NHS geriatric beds in England were closed. As a result elderly people, who had been cared for by nurses in hospital, were transferred to means-tested private accommodation. The rationale was to transfer costs from health service budgets to individuals, local authorities and the Social Security budget. Since 1994 health authorities have drawn up their own definitions of the people who should receive continuing health service care and those who should be transferred to private nursing homes. This means that a person in one area may qualify for free care, while in another area someone with identical needs will not. The changed role of the NHS in continuing care was never publicly debated. It was brought to public notice when there was an outcry from people of middle income (or their children) who were forced to sell their homes to pay for the costs of nursing care.

In other areas, public involvement is limited because there are no forums where people can engage in debate. Decisions about who receives health care and who does not, whether explicit or implicit, are essentially decisions about the value put on individual members of society. Without a national framework, inequalities in access to even basic services will develop across different areas. In some areas expensive new cancer drugs, continuing care or IVF may be available free, whereas in neighbouring areas they may not. One area may invest in mental health services, while a neighbouring area may not. Leaving rationing to undemocratic local health authorities to tackle within their funding constraints has political advantages because it does not implicate the government or politicians in unpopular decisions.

Medical research also throws up an increasing number of ethical issues. When does life begin: at what point does a foetus become a baby with rights? When does life end: at what point should someone in a persistent vegetative state be allowed to die? In what circumstances do people have the right to refuse to be treated, even if this will lead to their death? At present there tend to be short bursts of interest in the media about particular cases – about the 'mercy' killing of someone who is dying, the abortion of one foetus in a pregnancy with multiple embryos, or the treatment of an individual – such as a smoker who is refused heart surgery or a child refused cancer treatment. Debates about rationing and ethics focus on individual cases and interest is not sustained.

Often it is left to 'experts' to react, leaving little opportunity for public debate. In the UK, governments seem to respond to public concern by setting up ad hoc committees. In autumn 1997 two ad hoc committees were set up within two weeks of each other, both to do with the status of the human embryo: one on the use and storage of gametes (human reproductive cells) and another on surrogate pregnancies. There are also three different committees advising on human genetics. There is no national forum for general debates and this piecemeal approach does not encourage a wider debate or a coherent approach to ethical issues (Nicholson, 1997).

In some countries, there are national ethics committees that take a broader approach and can encourage public debate. There is an increasing consensus among professional and user bodies that a national ethics committee should be established to improve public visibility of medical ethics and ensure that the judgements made by local ethics committees are not covert or concealed (Benster and Pollock, 1993).

Professional interests

Though their power base has been undermined since the 1980s, professional groups and trade unions are well placed to bargain with government and to disrupt the implementation of policies with which they disagree. For example, the government needs the British Medical Association (BMA), as the representative of the medical profession, on its side to implement its policies. As experts, BMA members are also involved in advising the government on policy. In the history of the NHS many compromises have been made to accommodate the wish of doctors to maintain their independence and clinical freedom.

During the 1980s there were many cases of 'shroud waving' by professionals, unions and voluntary organizations. Publicity was given to individuals who were not receiving the treatment they needed, as part of campaigns for more resources for the NHS. The government response to these calls for more funding was to initiate the NHS review that led to the NHS and Community Care Act 1990, which changed the basis of the NHS. Health authorities and GP fundholders became purchasers in an internal market, with NHS and private providers competing for contracts from them.

Professional organizations and voluntary organizations worked together to resist the proposals for an internal health care market. Professional organizations have the resources to run public campaigns and to lobby ministers and government departments. In 1989 the BMA opposed the changes proposed in the White Paper, *Working for Patients*. In opposing the introduction of the internal health care market, the BMA ran a poster campaign against government policy in general and the Secretary of State, Kenneth Clarke, in particular. The posters appeared on hoardings all round the country and featured a photo of Kenneth Clarke with the heading: *'What do you call a man who ignores medical advice?'*. However, they were not as successful as they had been in the past. The government could afford in this instance to override the views of the medical profession, partly because the medical profession had lost some of its power to managers in the 1980s. Many doctors were under pressure by managers not to oppose their hospitals becoming NHS trusts. The threat used was that they would not be given funds to develop their own services if they opposed these plans (Butler, 1992).

Professionals may attempt to promote their specialty by influencing public opinion. The media and some obstetricians are promoting the right of women to have a Caesarean on demand without a medical reason, in spite of the risks this involves. 'Choice', which is an important consumer value, may be used to justify and promote more interventions and more medicalization of childbirth. In 1998 *Bella* magazine had an article 'Caesareans: should we be able to demand them?'. It had commissioned a survey in which women were asked if they thought that a woman should be able to opt for a Caesarean section without any medical reason. As part of the question respondents were told that some doctors had been arguing that planned Caesareans were safer than natural childbirth, but they were not told about the dangers of elective Caesareans. It is perhaps not surprising, therefore, that 47 per cent of women thought they should have this right. Women under 25 were more than twice as likely than women aged 45 to 54 to believe that Caesareans on demand were a good thing (Beech, 1998). Opinion polls can be used to give biased information and to promote particular points of view (Lohmann, 1998).

Professionals also share common interests with pharmaceutical companies in making new drugs available and may rely on them to fund research (Chapter 4). Pharmaceutical companies are great supporters of the right of doctors to exercise clinical freedom to prescribe whatever medicines they wish and not to be restricted on grounds of cost. Professionals can be effective lobbyists for pharmaceutical companies, particularly in their role as members of expert committees.

Industrial and commercial interests

Many industrial and commercial interests are concerned with influencing health policy. There are those representing commercial interests directly concerned with health care (such as private health services and pharmaceutical companies), which have benefited from decisions to deregulate health care and the encouragement of NHS and local authority purchasers to buy services from the private sector. The private sector also includes organizations which supply services to the NHS, such as cleaning, catering and laboratory services – organizations which have profited from the decision that health and local authorities must put services out to tender. The Public Finance Initiative enables commercial companies to build new hospitals and lease them back over many years to the NHS. This provides opportunities for long-term profits for investors.

Then there are those bodies representing commercial interests whose products or activities may – directly or indirectly – damage people's health, such as the tobacco and alcohol industries, and industries making products or using processes that pollute the environment. Stricter health and safety at work and environmental regulation will affect company profits, and so possibly jobs. There is also the road transport lobby that represents commercial interests and much of the public who want cheap motoring and are unwilling or unable to use public transport.

Companies spend a lot of money on public relations and lobbying. They are increasingly wanting to build partnerships and co-operate with public interest groups. However, this may be a PR strategy in order to maintain a favourable climate for business and a method of 'engineering consent' (Richter, 1998). Richter points out that the process has three main, sometimes overlapping components: intelligence gathering, manipulating public debate in a direction favourable to the company, and attempting to exclude what the industry perceives as diverging or antagonistic voices from public debates. Voluntary organizations need to be wary of requests from transnational companies to have a 'dialogue' or to 'co-operate' (Chapter 7).

The tobacco industry and the pharmaceutical and food industries illustrate how powerful the influence of commercial interests can be on health policy. The lobbying power of industry is also seen in the field of control of environmental hazards.

Tobacco industry

The ease with which commercial interests can obtain access to government can be illustrated in the success for the tobacco lobby that brought an end to the honeymoon for the new Labour Government in 1997. The Labour Party in its manifesto had included a Europe-wide ban on tobacco advertising which the previous Conservative Government had been blocking. In November 1997, the government announced the ban would be introduced but that sponsorship for Formula 1 motor racing would be exempt. The main reason given for the change in policy was the threat of a loss of jobs in the UK. Nevertheless, there was public cynicism as the decision followed a major donation by a businessman involved in Formula 1 to the Labour Party, along with revelations about the extent to which racing teams were sponsored by individual tobacco manufacturers.

Commercial interests often have a wide network of support in Parliament. They can persuade MPs to represent their interests by offering them paid consultancies and directorships or by offering them lavish hospitality. For example, in the 1980s it was estimated that about one hundred MPs actively supported the tobacco industry. They included MPs paid for parliamentary lobbying, MPs from constituencies where people were employed in the industry, or MPs involved in advertising or public relations companies that represented tobacco companies or firms such as newspapers and magazines that benefit from tobacco advertising

(Taylor, 1985). Often it is also the MPs with an interest in a particular area who get on to the government committees which are looking into that area. There is now a requirement for MPs to register their interests. This is a start, but declaring an interest does not always reduce influence or access to people who make decisions.

The tobacco industry funds organizations to campaign on its behalf, arguing on the grounds of consumer freedom and rights. FOREST (the Freedom Organization for the Right to Enjoy Smoking Tobacco) was launched in 1981 when the tobacco industry felt threatened by the then junior health minister, Sir George Young. He had strong views about the importance of reducing smoking and supported a total ban on tobacco advertising (Taylor, 1985). The purpose of FOREST is not to promote smoking, but to restore freedom of choice for: 'a group of people constantly forgotten, ignored, castigated, discriminated against and victimized: the adult consumer of tobacco products'.

Pharmaceutical industries

The British pharmaceutical industry is one of the most successful business operations in the UK. While most of UK manufacturing industry shrank in the late 1970s and 1980s, the number of people employed by drug companies gradually rose. Currently the number of staff employed in the UK by drug companies is around 75 000 with an additional 250 000 people employed indirectly as a consequence of the industry's activity. The UK pharmaceutical industry's trade surplus is now running at over £2.2 billion a year and is second only to that of the motor vehicle industry (Consumers' Association et al., 1997).

Pharmaceutical companies are, therefore, in a strong position to influence governments as major employers, exporters and contributors to the balance of trade surplus. Profits for pharmaceutical companies are guaranteed by the Pharmaceutical Price Regulation Scheme which agrees the profit margins allowed to companies by the Department of Health in the prices charged to the NHS. In addition, the Medicines Act 1968 guarantees them secrecy. Recently the power base of the pharmaceutical industry has been strengthened, through 'partnerships' with NHS providers to develop service packages for particular diseases, such as asthma and diabetes ('disease management'). Pharmaceutical companies see disease management as a way of increasing the use of drugs – by, for example, substituting drug therapy for other treatments. In the USA, pharmaceutical companies involved in disease management are extending their role beyond developing and producing drugs to also providing services. They fund projects in exchange for an exclusive supply agreement for their products. In Europe, the pharmaceutical industry is also promoting disease management as an approach, though more indirectly. In the UK and Europe disease management is seen as the way that services can be improved and costs contained at the same time, and is being developed through local initiatives (Rosleff and Lister, 1995). Disease management presents a dilemma for consumers. On the one hand it is attractive to have specialist care for your condition, in particular where other health services are being cut back. But on the other hand, it is not clear what the links will be between that company's products and the information it provides and what protection or choice there will be for users.

The food industry

Changes in eating habits, such as eating less sugars, salt and fat threaten both commercial profits and jobs. For example, the way that commercial interests conflict with those of health can be seen in the production and marketing of baby milk and infant food. While health professionals firmly support breastfeeding as best for mother and baby, manufacturers want to market and promote their baby milk formulas. Although the UK government supports the International Code of Marketing Breast-milk Substitutes, not all the requirements of the Code are included in UK law. For example, the International Code does not permit the promotion of any breast milk substitutes within health services or outside them. In the UK, however, breast milk substitutes can be promoted within the health service. Baby milk manufacturers can offer sponsorship and inducements to health workers, and contact mothers directly to promote their products. Companies often have a high profile at health conferences, including those run by the Royal College of Midwives. One NHS trust entered into a sponsorship deal, which gave midwives cardigans which had the sponsoring company's logo on them. These were withdrawn after complaints that this would be a breach of the International Code (Baby Milk Action, 1997a). Baby food manufacturers also run helplines that provide advice to parents. These cannot provide independent advice, though this is not clear in the promotional material.

Sweet food manufacturers also have lobbied successfully about nutritional standards and the national diet. The cardiovascular group of the government's Committee on Medical Aspects of Food Policy (COMA) prepared a draft report in 1993. It compared what was considered to be a healthy diet with what people actually purchased, as revealed in the National Food Survey. Though there was not a great gap, it did show that people needed to reduce the fat, sugars and salt they ate and increase the fruit and vegetables, in particular starches such as potatoes. The sweet food manufacturers saw the report before publication and were concerned about the recommendation that people should reduce sugars in their diet and held private meetings with ministers in an attempt to get the report changed or suppressed. The COMA report was leaked to the press in August 1994 and government was accused of setting up a nanny state and telling people what they had to eat. As a result of this, the government found it difficult to defend the COMA report without being accused of promoting a nanny state. The report was published in November 1994 after a well co-ordinated briefing of the media by the National Food Alliance that supported the COMA report (AIS, 1994). Turning a debate about public health to one about the freedom of the individual is a tactic that has also been used by the tobacco industry in campaigning against the anti-smoking lobby.

Environmental hazards

Commercial interests also lobby to limit regulations controlling environmental pollutants produced by industrial processes. Better measurement of pollutants and their effects on health, and more openness in regulatory bodies, could have serious implications for manufacturers. If it is accepted that much ill health and disease are due to industrial pollution, both in the workplace and in the environment, pressure would grow for more regulation of industries which expose workers and the public to damaging pollutants. In spite of awareness of the possible chronic effects of pollutants, there has been little or no research conducted to provide evidence that might lead to increased public pressure for stronger regulation.

For example, fine particles, the invisible soot from power plants, cars and lorries are major polluters. In the USA it is estimated that three per cent of all deaths are caused by air pollution from such combustion processes. There is also the long-term damage to health caused by reduced lung function, including asthma, hay fever and chronic respiratory diseases. In the UK there has been little measurement of the emissions or epidemiological surveys to look at the long-term effects of fine particle pollution (Watson, 1996).

Similarly, there has been little or no research to establish the incidence of chronic exposure to low level pesticides (Beaumont, 1993). Some pesticides, for example DDT and Dioxin, stimulate the body's production of oestrogen and this may lead to breast cancer. Dramatic data from Israel showed that deaths from breast cancer had been very high among younger women in Israel, but between 1976 and 1986 there was a sudden drop of 30 per cent in deaths of women under 44 years of age. The conclusion was that this was due to a ban on Lindane, DDT and benzene hexachloride in 1978 (Westin and Richter, 1990). Since then Lindane has also been banned in other countries, though not the UK.

Charities, voluntary organizations and user groups

In comparison to professional and commercial interests, the lobby for consumer or public interests is weak. The only sanction against the government the voluntary sector has is to influence public opinion and voters. Many voluntary organizations start out because the founders want to do something about a particular problem. They publicize and campaign for their cause. However, charities cannot be seen as 'political', according to charity law. Many charities tread a difficult legal balance in order to represent their members' concerns without appearing too 'political'.

There are many voluntary organizations involved in health at national level. Some are primarily fund-raising organizations for medical research or particular hospitals or services; others are primarily providers of services and self-help; yet others are campaigning and lobbying groups. The first advocates for many users were enlightened professionals or concerned citizens. Then parents became involved in setting up organizations to lobby for better services for their children and people with learning difficulties. Finally, users started to set up their own organizations and speak for themselves. In these organizations the experience of being or having been a user, rather than professional knowledge, is an essential part of the membership and constitutes the legitimacy of the organization. During the 1980s and 1990s there has been a rise of user-led organizations.

In looking at how campaigning is undertaken around health issues, it is important to look at who makes policy within voluntary organizations. Most voluntary organizations involve users, concerned citizens (lay people) and professionals, but the balance is crucial in determining how they work and the contribution they make in national debates. Organizations can be seen in three broad, but by no means rigid groups: professionally-led organizations, organizations where professionals and users work in partnership, and user-led groups. Organizations are dynamic and change; user-led groups may become 'professional' and start to work closely with sympathetic professionals, as they become more established. Organizations set up by professionals or concerned citizens may become user-led. This is summarized in Figure 6.1.

Professionally-led groups

The richest voluntary organizations are the research charities that were set up when the urgent need was medical research. Consequently the interests of professionals and users were identical. These include organizations such as the Imperial Cancer Campaign, the British Heart Foundation and the British Diabetic Association. Professionals tend to be heavily involved in these organizations which help them to raise funds and promote their specialty. The decisions about research funded by charities are generally decided by professionals, not users or lay people (Chapter 4).

The conflict that may arise between professional and user interests in the large professionally dominated organizations is illustrated by events following the introduction of genetically produced 'human' insulin. The initial research for 'human' insulin was undertaken by the chair of the British Diabetic Association (BDA) and it was introduced in 1982 to replace animal-based insulin. Between 1986 and 1989 the BDA received up to 3000 letters from people with diabetes or their carers describing serious side effects arising from the new form of insulin. People became

Main objectives/activities	Values	Comments	Examples
Professionally-led • Research • Support of professionals • Information to patients	Professional values and expertise dominate and give the organization its legitimacy	Large financial reserves Links with professional bodies and the commercial sector Users mainly involved in raising funds	British Diabetic Association British Heart Foundation Imperial Cancer Research Fund Mental Health Foundation
User and professional partnerships • Providing services • Self-help, information and support • Campaigning	Policies negotiated between users and professionals Legitimacy based on this balance	Funding from variety of sources, but may be short term without large reserves Users involved in all activities, often shared with sympathetic professionals Carers may be involved more than patients	Action for Sick Children National Childbirth Trust MIND Terrence Higgins Trust
User-led • Self-help, information and support • Campaigning	Experience of being a user valued above professional expertise and this gives the group its legitimacy	Patients may be involved more than carers Small with limited funds, often suspicious of funding tied to professional or commercial interests May be unstable, to survive they may become professionalized and become a partnership organization	AIMS Survivors Speak Out RAGE (Radiotherapy Action Group Exposure) People First

Figure 6.1 *Range of national organizations involved in health*
Note: These are idealized categories; the boundaries can shift and organizations move between groups at different stages of their development.

angry because neither their doctors nor the BDA believed that their symptoms were due to the new insulin. After a battle within the BDA, a Task Force was set up to look at the issue. Their report concluded the symptoms people reported were real, and that great distress and a break-down in doctor–patient relationships had been caused because patients were not believed. The BDA did not publish the report. As a result some members of the BDA left and set up a new organization, the Insulin Dependent Diabetes Trust. They believed that the close links between professionals, researchers and the pharmaceutical companies meant that organizations such as the BDA were unable to represent their interests any longer (Hirst, 1997).

Some professionally-led organizations, like the British Diabetic Association, were set up to fight disease. Others are set up to lobby against trends which threaten particular interests, such as HealthWatch (formerly the Campaign Against Health Fraud) which was set up in 1989 in the UK. The aims were laudable, as outlined in *The Times* newspaper on 8 May 1989: 'promoting assessments of new treatments and protecting con-sumers from fraudulent claims. It will act as an independent information service for journalists who want to comment on fraud in medicine'. HealthWatch campaigns for orthodox medicine against complementary and alternative practitioners, often very effectively. Membership is largely from among orthodox clinicians and it has close links with the pharma-ceutical industry. It has never been or tried to be a consumer-based organization (Walker, 1993). HealthWatch was based on the American National Council Against Health Fraud which was set up in 1984 to campaign against unorthodox medicine. It was the US gay community who first demonstrated against the National Council Against Health Fraud. They objected to an organization that wanted to stop them trying alternative treatments when the only orthodox treatment available for them was AZT, which not everyone could take.

User and professionals partnerships

Some groups may be set up by professionals or users who are frustrated by orthodox approaches. For example, the Coronary Prevention Group was set up in 1979 by doctors who were critical of the approach of the British Heart Foundation. They believe that coronary heart disease is a disease of poverty rather than simply being caused by diet and lifestyle, and they work closely with voluntary groups. The Public Health Alliance, set up in 1987, is made up of professionals, trade unions and voluntary bodies; it is committed to promoting public health and has an advocacy role in counterbalancing powerful commercial interests. The Association for Public Health was set up in 1992 as a professionally led organization – an alternative, more establishment public health organization that was more willing to work with government than the Public Health Alliance. By 1998, with a government prepared to talk about inequalities and social justice, a merger was proposed between the two groups as many felt that the split weakened the public health movement. Others feared that the radical agenda of the Public Health Alliance would be lost with the merger (Millar, 1998).

Other voluntary organizations are set up by users in partnership with sympathetic professionals to promote better services, often in line with government policies. Voluntary organizations are often in a good position to campaign against inertia in local services or to undertake tasks which professions or government find politically too sensitive to do themselves. The Department of Health gives grants to national voluntary organizations to promote government policy; these organizations include those such as Action for Smoking and Health (ASH), which support health education programmes, and more service-oriented organizations such as MIND, MENCAP and Age Concern. Too much reliance on government and short-term funding may inhibit voluntary organizations in the way that they put forward the views of their members, since their funding often depends on accepting national policy.

An example of an organization that is 'shared' between users and professionals is Action for Sick Children. It was set up in 1961 as Mother Care in Hospital by a group of mothers who wanted to stay with their sick children in hospital. At that time visiting was restricted in hospital and nurses found that children did not cry or seem to get upset if their parents did not visit. Staff did not realize that what they saw as a 'good' child was, in fact, a withdrawn child, often in a state of shock, who was at risk of long-term emotional damage. Since the *Platt Report* in 1959, Department of Health policy has been that a parent should be admitted to hospital with their child. Mother Care in Hospital became the National Association for the Welfare of Children in Hospital and then Action for Sick Children. It encourages professionals to work as partners with parents in the care of their children and campaigns for separate, child-friendly services which employ staff with specialized training to work with children. Professionals sympathetic to its aims are involved in the management of the organization and in supervising projects.

One of the most well-informed and apparently effective user lobbies has been for maternity services. Maternity services are different from most other health services since women are generally in good health. After the first baby, women usually know what to expect and what they want. Until the NHS was established in 1948 most women gave birth at home with the help of a midwife. Then obstetricians became involved and most births took place in hospital. Childbirth, hitherto a normal event with risks, became a medical event involving interventions, tests and technology. Women began to challenge doctors. The Natural Childbirth Association, later the National Childbirth Trust (NCT), was set up in 1956 to promote the ideas of a radical doctor, Grantly Dick-Read. The NCT was committed to birth either at home or in homely, non-threatening maternity units. At that time it took enormous courage to raise these matters in public.

Pregnancy and birth were taboo subjects and the NCT was criticized by the BMA and the public on the grounds of 'good taste' (Moorhead, 1996). Though the NCT challenged obstetric care, some of the key figures in the organization had a medical background and the NCT has continued to co-operate with professionals.

In spite of the fact that user organizations have been successful in influencing national policies and largely campaign for the implementation of government policies, they have not had the success that might have been expected. Nearly forty years later, most children's services are child-friendly and welcome parents, but many children are still admitted to adult wards that do not have specially trained staff or facilities for them (Action for Sick Children (Scotland), 1995). In childbirth, unlike most other areas, user representatives are accepted as 'experts'. As such they may be represented on national 'expert' committees and lay people are expected, where possible, to take the chair of local multi-disciplinary maternity services liaison committees. In 1993 the views of AIMS and the NCT were accepted in a report, *Changing Childbirth*, which proposed changes to maternity services which would mean that each woman would have more choice and control over her labour and delivery (Department of Health, 1993). In spite of this, interventions in childbirth have not decreased (Chapter 4). It seems that there are even more powerful professional and commercial interests working against this initiative.

User-led organizations

An example of a user-led organization is the Association for Improvements in Maternity Services (AIMS) which was set up in 1960 as the Society for the Prevention of Cruelty to Pregnant Women. It took a different approach from the NCT which had been set up a few years earlier. Members defined childbirth as a normal event, which in effect meant that there were no areas of expertise where the views of 'lay' people could be discounted. Complaints from women about, for example, problems caused by induction, led AIMS to go back to the research literature. They were surprised by what they found. Jean Robinson reports her experience in the 1970s:

> One of the first papers I read was a randomized trial in *The Lancet* apparently designed to prove that elective induction at term would reduce the incidence of mature stillbirth. It proved nothing of the kind, and what is more the references and authors quoted to show induction was safe, in fact said the reverse. (Robinson, 1995)

AIMS has not had the same support from professionals as the NCT. It criticizes individual hospitals that it considers are failing women. It has not attempted to obtain funding except from subscriptions and its members.

Mental health organizations that have been set up by users and those set up by professionals and carers often have different views. Survivors Speak Out was set up in 1986 by people who felt that they had been abused by the mental health system. Survivors Speak Out wants less coercion, fewer in-patient facilities, more social support and help in ordinary environments. In contrast, the National Schizophrenia Fellowship and SANE (Schizophrenia A National Emergency) identify more with the views of parents and carers than those of patients. They tend to focus on the need for hospital beds and more control over patients. In 1987 they supported a campaign by the Royal College of Psychiatrists to modify the 1983 Mental Health Act to extend Compulsory Treatment Orders into the community, which would mean that psychiatrists would have the legal right to force people to take medication while living in the community. Opposing this were MIND and Survivors Speak Out. A campaign by SANE worked on public prejudice and fears; they used a poster to campaign against community care that said: 'He thinks he is Jesus. You think he's a killer. They think he is fine' (Rogers et al., 1993).

Voluntary organizations for people with HIV and AIDS have demonstrated what can be done if people work together. In the late 1980s and early 1990s there was considerable funding available for HIV and AIDS, and many organizations were set up to provide support for people who were HIV positive and services for people with AIDS. The work of HIV activists in the 1980s gave a great boost to the hospice movement and pointed to the importance of social conditions, such as housing, social support and income for people living with HIV. HIV organizations became politically active in campaigning for resources for people with the condition and have been successful in maintaining funding for drug treatments for people with AIDS. Their example has been important in encouraging groups representing people with other conditions to become more politically active. However, within HIV organizations there have been tensions between people who are HIV positive and people who have not been tested for HIV. Some, like Positively Women, started out as a self-help group but later decided to employ untested women in order to develop and expand its services.

Even the most vulnerable people are setting up their own organizations. The first organization of, as opposed to for, people with learning difficulties was called People First and was set up in the 1970s in Oregon, USA. In 1996 an organization was set up within the National Children's Bureau to enable children to represent themselves directly. It was named Article 12 after the article in the UN Convention on the Rights of the Child which safeguards the rights of children and young people to express their opinions. Members are aged between 5 and 17 years. The steering committee is made up of children and young people with the help of an adult support worker. However, there are difficulties for the more vulnerable user-led groups who have to rely on advisers. Dowson (1990: 3) points out that people with learning difficulties are at a particular disadvantage in learning who to trust: 'How difficult it is to choose your allies when you are reliant on your allies to advise you!' Funding for voluntary organizations often depends on accepting orthodoxy – whether the orthodoxy of professionals, the government or the pharmaceutical industry. Some user groups have taken over territory generally considered to be that of experts and clinicians, and challenge the establishment and professionally dominated charities – but they have difficulty obtaining funding. The lack of funding may mean that they are unstable and vulnerable to illness or 'burn-out' of key activists. Some may become 'partnership' organizations in order to achieve stability and become established. User-led pressure groups that, almost by definition, do not accept conventional views about what they need and how services should be provided for them, may be easily dismissed. In order to be heard, they may need to broaden their campaigns to wider social issues and make alliances with other groups – such as the environmental, disability and anti-poverty lobbies – in order to have a stronger voice.

'Partnerships' with commercial companies

While charities have long-established links with professionals, links with commercial companies are more recent. Both drug companies and voluntary organizations are now recognizing the common ground they share. Many patients depend on a wide range of medicines being available. This was highlighted in 1985 when the Department of Health introduced a limited list of pharmaceutical products that would be available on the NHS. It was patient representatives who acted to prevent the blacklisting of medicines they wanted, especially for skin conditions and oral contraceptives. As 'partners' with pharmaceutical companies, voluntary organizations can get access to funding, information and policy makers through these links.

There are great advantages for drug companies in dealing directly with patients. Initially the company may obtain good public relations and advertising by being associated in the minds of patients and professionals with feel-good initiatives. In the long run they may be able to bypass medical professionals, who may be more sceptical and conscious of costs. By supporting voluntary organizations, pharmaceutical companies can help create consumer demand for their drugs and exert pressure to fast track a drug through the licensing procedures. Once it is licensed, user groups can lobby to ensure that their members know about the new drug and lobby to make it widely available. The Multiple Sclerosis Society campaigned in the 1990s to ensure that beta interferon is available. HIV and AIDS organizations have been active in publicizing and creating pressures on health authorities to make new but expensive combination drug therapies available.

There are shared interests between drug companies and voluntary organizations in some areas, but the links that the organization has to professional or commercial groups may influence the issues on which it campaigns. For example, the pharmaceutical company, Wellcome, dominated the AIDS scene from 1987. It had developed the only licensed AIDS drug and funded many HIV organizations in the late 1980s and early 1990s. The Terrence Higgins Trust, the most important organization providing information and advice on HIV and AIDS, was unambiguous in its promotion of AZT as the best treatment – even to the extent of pursuing complaints to the General Medical Council against doctors working on nutrition-based therapies. In 1992 the Terrence Higgins Trust produced a series of expensively produced booklets about HIV and AIDS which were apparently written with the help of Wellcome. These were criticized for presenting a selective view of HIV infection and its treatment which meant they were a sophisticated form of advertising for Wellcome (Walker, 1993).

As a further example, when there was publicity about serious side effects of a drug commonly used for acne, the manufacturer's first move was to start to fund an acne support group – as reported in *Private Eye* on 6 March 1998. The issue of the group's newsletter following this had an article by its chair, who was a consultant dermatologist. He accused the media of creating a scare. However, some people were angry that they had experienced side effects for two years, including lupus and hepatitis, which were not recognized as due to the drug. Some of them are taking legal action against the pharmaceutical company.

Difficulties in raising independent funding mean that the pressure to survive in a difficult climate has persuaded many voluntary organizations to accept commercial funding. Concerns about conflicts of interest may cause divisions within the organization and lead to splits among members. This happened in 1997 when the National Childbirth Trust (NCT) for the first time accepted funding from a manufacturer of baby milk and baby foods. This led to the resignation of 70 of its voluntary breastfeeding counsellors and tutors who left to start a new organization – the Breastfeeding Network – which could offer independent information and support for breastfeeding mothers. They felt that the NCT was no longer able to do this (Baby Milk Action, 1997b).

A relationship between such a powerful group as the pharmaceutical industry and such a relatively weak group as users, can hardly be called a partnership. In the long term such 'partnerships' are so unequal in the access to power and resources that the voluntary sector may lose its credibility and independence (see Chapter 8 on the myth of patients as partners).

Co-ordinating the voice for users

There are several organizations representing health service users in general, rather than people with a specific condition or users of particular services. However, the views of the public and users on wider issues affecting health are not well co-ordinated. This means that the influence users have on general national policies is weak.

In 1974 the government recognized the need for a strong national voice for users. It proposed that a national council of CHCs should be set up which would draw on the experiences of CHCs but be independent of them. However, CHCs were suspicious and wanted a national organization that they could control, not one imposed on them by the Labour Government. As a result, the Association of Community Health Councils for England and Wales (ACHCEW) was set up by statute as a membership organization for CHCs. Though it can draw on the wide network of member CHCs, by its constitution it must reach a consensus among CHCs, which are politically and socially diverse. As a result it is limited in what it can say or do (Hogg, 1989).

If CHCs have been unable to provide the strong national voice for users, neither have other organizations. General user bodies include the National Consumer Council, which was set up by government to represent the interests of consumers, and the independent Consumers' Association which provides information on value for money of competing goods and services. There are also organizations concerned with general health issues, such as the Patients' Association and the College of Health. Those organizations concerned with general health issues contribute to national debates but they also generally have limited grass-roots user or public membership.

Voluntary organizations involved with health do not, in general, work closely together. Coalitions to encourage co-operation have had limited success, though this may be changing. The Patients' Forum, run for some years by the Patients' Association, did not move beyond a forum for sharing information and experiences. Since 1990 there have been more alliances between organizations to share good practice and also to lobby for the voluntary sector and its users. Umbrella groups and alliances such as the Long-Term Medical Conditions Alliance and the Disability Network have been set up. These alliances may be increasingly important as the advocacy role of the voluntary sector is limited as sources of funding become tied to contracts.

There are many reasons for this lack of a co-ordinated voice for users. First, most people who want to get involved in health issues either become involved with groups representing their specific interest or do so through professional organizations or trade unions. There is more satisfaction and likelihood of success in campaigning for their particular cause, since on broader issues of health policy they are less likely to have an influence: their expertise is more limited and there are other more powerful players.

Secondly, the voluntary sector is so diverse that even organizations with common concerns may find it difficult to sustain a co-ordinated lobby. Furthermore they may be competing for funding with others in the same field who have a different slant on the same problem. The World Cancer Research Fund, for example, concentrates on preventing cancer by persuading people to change their diet and lifestyle. The Women's National Cancer Control Campaign focuses on campaigns to raise awareness of the importance of regular cervical smears and breast awareness. Environmental contributions to the causes of cancer are not given much attention by either group. It has been the Women's Environmental Network that has taken this up, working with individuals and communities to map the incidence of breast cancer alongside sources of pollution – funded by the National Lottery. While all three approaches are valid, diversity may weaken the messages that organizations do agree about and give a one-sided view of the issues involved in preventing cancers.

Thirdly, the activities individual voluntary groups can undertake depend on what funds they raise. The funding they have may depend on undertaking particular projects, accepting government policies, or linking their activities to the interests of a better resourced and more powerful group. Most do not have the funds to give priority to campaigns or collaboration and networking, particularly if it is likely to antagonize its other funders.

Fourthly, voluntary groups may be 'captured' by more powerful organizations, whether governmental, professional or commercial. For any group that has not been consulted before, it is flattering to be recognized and consulted, especially if it has been campaigning for a long time for this. More powerful interests can use flattery and funding to divide voluntary organizations and lessen the impact of their message; sometimes voluntary organizations seem to be better at making alliances with professional or commercial interests than with each other.

Strength as a pressure group rests in making alliances to lobby decision makers. There is a need for an independent co-ordinated lobby for users, building on the common ground that groups coming from different perspectives share. The importance of a strong independent user voice at national level has been recognized in the Netherlands and in Australia. In 1981 the Dutch government published a policy document about improving the position of patients in health care. Following this, the national federation of patient and consumer organizations was set up as a coalition of consumer organizations, patients' organizations and organizations of elderly people. About 1.7 million people are organized within these bodies which means that between fifteen and twenty per cent of the adult population is organized in some way around aspects of health care. Before the coalition was set up, the user lobby was scattered and ineffective in the Netherlands. The government supported the coalition because it was a way of bringing some equity between professionals, third-party payers, consumers and other interests (Dekkers, 1995). The coalition provides information to give users more freedom of choice; defines the needs of patients through surveys and research; co-ordinates the strategies of interest groups, integrating both citizens' and users' views and, finally, promotes the implementation of patients' rights.

Similarly, Australia has established a consumer health forum to provide the minister of health with an early and coherent voice from community and consumer organizations. The forum is made up of health, social service, consumer, environmental, ethnic, women's and pensioners' groups. It is intended as a counterbalance to the strong vested interests of medical and industrial groups (Milo, 1988). The forum disseminates information on available training and research funds; designs research projects; monitors progress towards greater community participation: and promotes public understanding of policy decisions. The forum is mostly funded by government and is co-ordinated by a core of 16 community organizations with an elected executive committee.

Health interest groups could gain further strength from linking up with wider groups that share common concerns, particularly in lobbying against commercial interests that damage health. There is increasing political activity outside mainstream politics in organizations described as 'social movements'. These include the women's movement, the peace movement and the environmental lobby. Their prime objective is to get issues and ideas onto the political agenda. They tend to be looser and more informal than traditional interest groups and use direct action rather than mainstream politics to further their cause (Byrne, 1997).

Conclusions

At a national level, public interests are often marginalized by more powerful interests where commercial lobbies may work against the development of healthy public policies. The first requirement for involving the public is to reduce the secrecy in the way the government works. Greater public scrutiny and involvement would lead to more open decision making, which in turn generally results in better decisions.

Secondly, it is essential to recognize the value of the participation of users and citizens, and the importance of conflict and dissent in the democratic process. The reverence for the 'expert' in health services means that it is easy to exclude and undervalue their contributions or manipulate them to suit other interests. There is a need for arrangements to enable the public to contribute to debates, such as on ethics and rationing.

Thirdly, public funds need to be invested to ensure that there is a strong independent user movement. Only by having independent resources will the voluntary sector be able to maintain its credibility. Voluntary organizations that are funded by pharmaceutical companies will lose the ability to speak for many users. The lack of independence and competition for funding also divides the user movement, ultimately weakening its impact and undermining the representation of user views at national level.

In the past the rich charities were those that had the support and patronage of the most powerful group at the time, the professional establishment. In the future the richest charities may well be those that have the support and funding of the pharmaceutical companies. Alternative groups may be set up that see the commercial interests as a part of the cause of their problems, not the solution to them. Unfortunately, as with groups that have rejected professional orthodoxy, they will have difficulties in obtaining funding. To make an impact such organizations will need to develop wider alliances with other lobbies, such as those on civil rights, poverty, disability, race and the environment.

7

GLOBAL CITIZENS

Health for all will be achieved by people themselves.

World Health Organization, *Alma Ata Declaration* (1977)

The earth is one, but the world is not.

Brundtland Report (1987)

More and more our lives are affected by what happens overseas. We share the same planet and, increasingly, the same marketplace with citizens of other countries. National governments can no longer act by themselves to tackle the new threats to public health. For example, a nuclear disaster in Chernobyl in the Ukraine caused by poor maintenance, has had long-term effects on farmers in Wales, Scotland and the North of England. Even the climate is changing because of global warming which may mean that infectious diseases that until now have only been found in tropical climates will move north. Infectious diseases are re-emerging as a major health problem and they can quickly pass over borders. In 1946 the Constitution of the World Health Organization recognized the common dangers of unequal development in different countries of health promotion and control of disease, especially communicable disease. These trends are leading to more international regulation of health and safety, food processing, agriculture and the environment. With more world trade, safety standards for imports need to be internationally agreed; it is pointless having high standards for food safety in the UK if imported food can be sold which does not meet these standards and costs less to buy.

As citizens and users, it is no longer enough to lobby national governments: representation is needed at international level and in supranational policy making. Several international agencies, directly or indirectly, affect health in the UK – particularly those organizations whose rulings are mandatory on member countries, such as the European Union (EU) and the World Trade Organization. Other agencies such as the World Health Organization (WHO), the Organization for Economic Co-operation and Development (OECD), the World Bank and the Food and Agriculture

Organization (FAO) have some influence on policies. This chapter looks at how the policies of international agencies affect health care and public health policies in the UK, and how public interest and user groups try to participate in and influence international policies and decisions.

The consumer and user lobby

International agencies work with governments and so how far non-governmental organizations (NGOs) are involved depends on each national government's willingness to involve them. It also depends on the nature of the activities of the international agency. WHO, for example, needs the support of NGOs to implement its strategy of Health For All, whereas the OECD and the World Trade Organization are concerned with economic issues and trade for which they require the co-operation of commercial interests, but not public interest NGOs.

It has been estimated that there are about five hundred organizations and three thousand lobbyists centred around the European Union (EU). However, voluntary organizations comprise about only one per cent of them (Harvey, 1991). In contrast, commercial interests have been lobbying international and global institutions to their advantage for some time (Baine et al., 1992). There are difficulties for consumer organizations in campaigning together at an international level for two main reasons: the way international agencies operate and the problems in mobilizing NGOs at international level, including the seemingly eternal difficulties in obtaining independent funding.

NGOs have found it hard to be involved in the European Union because of the complex and bureaucratic way that decisions are made. Decision-making powers lie with the European Commission and the Council of Ministers who are required to consult Parliament, but are not compelled to take any action afterwards. The main role of the European Parliament is not to make laws but as a forum for debating values, directions and priorities in Europe. However, the power of the Parliament is increasing and can now veto budgets proposed by the Commission.

The President of the Commission and the Commissioners are not elected but nominated by national governments. The Commission initiates proposals for legislation, budgets and programmes of work. It also administers programmes and monitors the way in which the treaties and subsequent legislation are observed by member states. As health is not central to the EU, decisions about public health and consumer protection are made by different directorates with different agendas. Food and agriculture, industrial policy, environmental policy, transport policy, employment, social care, education and public health are all the responsibility of separate directorates. As a result health issues may involve many directorates. Policies on drug misuse, for example, involve justice, home affairs, youth and social policies directorates.

Another major difficulty for consumer and user groups is the secrecy with which many agencies operate, in particular the European Commission and the World Trade Organization. This is justified on the grounds that many discussions are about trade and tariffs which are traditionally confidential for commercial reasons. The Council of Ministers is the only legislative body in Europe that makes decisions in secret. The lack of transparency in the EU was tested when Sweden became a member. Sweden has had a Freedom of Information Act since 1766, under which people can now apply for EU documents. The Swedish Union of Journalists' newspaper applied, under Swedish law, for a set of 20 EU documents on Europol (Europe's new police agency) and were given 18 of them. When similar applications were made directly to the EU, only 4 out of the 20 documents were disclosed. Sweden has been accused of breaking community law because of its Freedom of Information Act. It is not yet clear whether Sweden's membership of the EU will increase transparency in Europe or restrict freedom of information in Sweden (Frankel, 1996).

In addition to the problem of the structure and accountability of international agencies, there are the difficulties in organizing and funding NGOs at an international level. Individual organizations from a single country carry little weight with international agencies. So in 1960 the International Organisation of Consumer Unions was set up to link consumer organizations across national borders. It changed its name to Consumers International in 1995 and has five regional offices and a membership of more than two hundred and twenty consumer groups in a hundred countries. Its mission has been to 'strive for a fairer society through defending the rights of consumers everywhere. In particular, Consumers International aims to protect the rights of the poor, the marginalised and the disadvantaged'.

In Europe representation at the European Commission is handled by the Bureau Européen des Unions de Consummateurs. The European Union first introduced a consumer policy in 1972 when it set up a consumer consultative committee with representatives of European consumer organizations. More and more European networks are being set up. Some are funded by the EC, perhaps because they provide an easier contact point than negotiating with individual countries. The European Public Health Alliance, a broad coalition of health groups based in Brussels, provides the secretariat for the Health Intergroup of MEPs in the European Parliament and lobbies international bodies. It is particularly concerned with monitoring EC activities that affect health, including health aspects of the Common Agricultural Policy.

Users with particular health conditions have much in common and are increasingly working internationally. People living with HIV and AIDS have been strongly represented at international biennial conferences held since the 1980s. The presence of activists in conferences normally only attended by scientists, clinicians and policy makers changed the content of conferences and created pressure for action. People living with HIV in the West have gained strength and influence in working internationally, though their concerns are very different from those of people in developing countries. In the West a major issue is ensuring access to expensive combination drug therapies, whereas people living with HIV in other countries may not even have access to food or money. For them, more important issues are HIV prevention and care for the children left orphaned.

The example of the HIV activists has inspired women with breast cancer to see their situation as a political and a feminist issue. Women started to question why breast cancer seemed to be regarded as a success story while more and more women were dying of it. Treatment that was unproved in its efficacy, but was known to be toxic, was given to women, while little research was undertaken into the environmental causes of breast cancer. The First International Conference on Breast Cancer Advocacy was held in 1997 in Brussels. More than two hundred and fifty breast cancer survivors, health professionals and consumer advocates from 11 countries met to talk about their experiences.

The European Patients' Voice was formed in 1998 to represent people who suffer from genetic disorders and might benefit from biotech patenting. The Cochrane Collaboration, which started in Oxford, provides a basis for enabling users to have a voice in clinical discussions internationally. The Collaboration is an international organization that aims to help people make well-informed decisions about health by preparing and maintaining systematic reviews of the benefits and risks of health care interventions. The work for the reviews is undertaken by groups, bringing together professionals and patient groups from several countries. Because the reviews focus on specific conditions, it is easy for patient groups to participate. There are now over a dozen centres around the world.

While most consumer groups, such as Consumers International, recognize the dangers of accepting commercial sponsorship, some patient groups, at international as well as national level, do not always share the view that there may be a conflict of interest between them and commercial – mainly pharmaceutical – companies. International seminars and conferences of self-help groups are often funded by pharmaceutical companies. In 1998 a new international alliance of patient organizations was set up with drug company sponsorship.

Health Action International believes that any drug company sponsorship of a health group or facility compromises the principle that consumers have the right to receive independent and objective information; thus, industry funding is not in the public's interest (Hayes and Mintzes, 1997). The European Public Health Alliance has produced guidelines for NGOs on accepting industry sponsorship (EPHA, 1995). However, these guidelines only work if industry-sponsored organizations apply them critically. Health Action International has suggested that such groups might consider having their publications and information services critically assessed by an outside organization that is independent of industry. While there are many areas of shared interest between NGOs and commercial organizations, the case against accepting commercial funding may be even stronger at international than at national level. One of the most important reasons for user groups to work together is the need to counterbalance the power of the transnationals and they will be limited in what they can do if they are funded by them.

The health care market

The development of an international health care market is leading to pressures to harmonize clinical standards, professional regulation and protection for victims of medical accidents. The EU works on the principle of 'subsidiarity' – the idea that decision making occurs at the lowest level possible in order to retain accountability. However, in health policy what is appropriate to national governments and what to the EU has not been defined. What is more, it is not clear how these should be defined.

There are several reasons why there are pressures towards harmonization in health care. First, regulations on the packaging and marketing of pharmaceuticals need to be standardized as part of a common market. Secondly, where patients and workers travel to other European countries, they need access to health care in these countries. Thirdly, as professionals cross borders to work in different countries their qualifications need to be internationally recognized. Finally, as research about drugs is carried out in centres in different countries, regulations need to be standardized and this brings in ethical considerations.

'Harmonization' of health care is complex because of cultural differences in clinical practice. Lynn Payer (1990), in her book *Medicine and Culture*, traced these differences. In France health problems tend to be attributed to the liver, in Germany to the heart and in England to the bowels. Many diseases result from an interaction between outside agents and the body's response. In the UK and the USA the main concern is with the outside agent (such as the bacterium or virus), whereas in France and Germany doctors are concerned with the internal factors which make an individual susceptible to illness. For this reason it is common for patients to be prescribed vitamins, tonics and spa treatment in France and Germany, but not in the UK or USA. In France and Germany there is much greater acceptance of homeopathy and what, in England, are regarded as fringe medicines. Antibiotics make up a smaller proportion of the medicines prescribed in France and Germany and doses of medicines tend to be less aggressive than in the UK or the USA.

European countries also organize and fund health care in different ways, varying from the insurance-based schemes of France and Germany to the publicly funded schemes of the UK and the Netherlands. These differences are reducing as an internal health care market develops and the same preoccupations – cost containment and the search for efficiency – dominate health policy in all Western countries.

Pharmaceutical products

An important area of harmonization of health care is in access to, and regulation of, pharmaceutical and health products. A single market requires standardization of pack sizes, dosages and names of drugs – all of which vary between countries. Medicines are treated as consumer goods and fall within the Single European Act which came into operation in 1987. They come under the EC Directorate dealing with competition. Because pharmaceutical products are treated as consumer goods, their production and regulation are not seen as public health issues and consultation with health organizations is, therefore, limited. However, clinical issues are involved as different dosages are prescribed for the same condition by practitioners in different countries. In France the standard insulin dose is less than half that used in the UK. This makes for complex calculations for diabetics who travel around Europe (NCC, 1991).

In many countries the most important issue for consumer groups is access to essential medicines and their safety. About one half of the world's population lacks access to essential medicines. In almost all developing countries the private sector controls the major share of the pharmaceutical market and their position is getting stronger. Recently the World Trade Organization extended the patent protection on medicines and this means that there will be delays to the introduction of cheaper generic drugs; so more drugs will be kept out of the reach of many people for a long time (HAI, 1997). Transnational pharmaceutical companies also oppose the development of local pharmaceutical manufacturing (Garrett, 1994).

Consumers often pay high prices for drugs that are unsafe or of little or no benefit (Heide, 1996). For example, before the political changes in Poland in 1989 there were drugs shortages but now there are too many drugs, many of which are obsolete, ineffective, expensive or potentially harmful. Consumers and health professionals had difficulty getting information and were under great pressure from aggressive and unethical drug promotions. A Polish consumer group, in association with Health Action International, undertook a campaign for the rational use of drugs. Though some drugs had been withdrawn by the government, consumer groups felt that the Polish government was more concerned with the local production of drugs than with safety for consumers (Skrzpiec, 1996). There are similar problems in the Ukraine where pharmaceuticals were brought into the country by private companies and sold through private pharmacies. The state was unable to establish strict control over imported medicines. Any attempts to do so met with resistance from the transnational pharmaceutical companies. The World Bank supported the pharmaceutical companies and its loans are conditional on the Ukraine's abolition of compulsory certification of imported drugs (Popova, 1996).

Though drugs are widely promoted and advertised, independent information is difficult for both the public and professionals to find in many countries. There are advantages for users of sharing information about pharmaceuticals and their side effects and co-operating internationally. For example, in the 1980s, people with diabetes in the UK who believed the new form of 'human' insulin was causing them severe side effects found that the same problems were being experienced by people in other countries, in particular in Switzerland where the drug had been introduced over a relatively short time as in the UK. In other countries where the introduction was slower, problems were slow to come to public attention. By sharing information, people with insulin dependent diabetes in other countries were alerted to possible side effects and the position of users in all countries was strengthened.

There are changes within pharmaceutical companies themselves that make international regulation even more important: the growing international mail-order market for drugs which bypasses national borders and regulations. A new system for regulating medicines in Europe was introduced in 1995 when the European Agency for the Evaluation of Medicinal Products (EMEA) was established in London. From January 1998, pharmaceutical companies can register their products though a central procedure in the Agency or by a 'mutual recognition procedure' which is run by national agencies. The Agency will deal with disputes about mutual recognition between countries. For innovative products and products derived from biotechnology, the Committee for Proprietary Medicinal Products (CPMP) decides about registration. Each country can nominate two members to serve on the committee, but there is no consumer representation and consumer organizations do not have observer status either.

Nevertheless the Agency has been concerned about transparency and provides access to documents, including access through the Internet. In response to a consultation on transparency and access to information the EMEA carried out in 1997, Health Action International pointed out that the information available fell short of what consumers needed and that evaluating medicines is a public health issue, and so consultation should not be restricted to consumer groups and the pharmaceutical industry (EMEA, 1997). The National Consumer Council in the UK has recommended that all information should be openly available unless it can be proved that disclosure would infringe a company's commercial rights, and that consumer representatives should be appointed to the CPMP (NCC, 1994b).

Over the past decade – through mergers, acquisitions and strategic alliances in the pharmaceutical industry – the top ten companies have increased their share of the market and are extending their activities into other areas of health care. They are acquiring companies which provide health care and which can be used as outlets for their products. In this way they can directly monitor patients' needs and influence what drugs are authorized. These trends could put up the costs of pharmaceutical products and put pharmaceutical companies in a stronger position to influence governments and international agencies (Kanavos, 1996). Public scrutiny of the activities of transnational pharmaceutical companies is increasingly important.

Patients travelling to other countries

Citizens of the European Union may go to another EU country for specialist treatments that are not available in their own country, or because the waiting lists are shorter. In future patients may be on a waiting list around a network of highly specialized hospitals in several countries. Already the Netherlands and Denmark fund patients to go to hospitals in other countries. Many London teaching hospitals attract patients from all over the world. These hospitals' survival may depend on attracting more patients in need of specialist treatment and expanding overseas trade (Akehurst, 1992). In the private sector, health care is increasingly provided by international hospital chains. BUPA operate in Spain and Ireland as well as the UK. The French chain, Vivendi, owns 18 institutions in England through the American Medical International. Cross-boundary travel by patients is still relatively low. But it is likely to rise so purchasers and insurance companies are looking at the implications of the international market (Leidl and Rhodes, 1997).

In theory an international health care market offers patients more choice. However, in the UK people have tended to be referred to regional or national specialist centres if they live nearby rather than on the basis of their clinical need for the specialist treatment (Hogg, 1992). In fact the development of an international health care market may adversely affect health services available for local people and divert resources from primary and community services, particularly in London. Eileen O'Keefe (1993) points out that this may have already affected the way that maternity services have developed in Central London. For several years it has been apparent that the pressing need in many areas of London is to develop a comprehensive community-based maternity service. However, obstetric services are still based in hospitals rather than community services, and staff have been appointed with expertise in high-tech areas of obstetrics and gynaecology with an eye on markets abroad.

Another implication of an international health care market is the need for shared regulatory systems and better methods of exchanging information about professionals who have been found guilty of serious professional misconduct. Regulatory systems at present vary between European countries. For example, the regulation of complementary practitioners varies from almost no regulation in the UK to tight regulation in France, Spain and Italy (Fisher and Ward, 1994).

Ethics and research

As the international market in health care and research develops, so ethical issues arise about the rights of patients. Countries have different cultural norms, political traditions, religions and lifestyles and so attempting 'convergence' or consensus on some ethical issues such as euthanasia or abortion is probably impossible. But there are issues where consensus is important. For example, agreeing a definition of when someone is dead is important in determining what organs are available for transplantation and has implications for the trade in human organs. In most countries, including the UK, patients or their relatives must state their willingness to donate organs. But in some countries, such as Belgium, it is assumed that they are willing to donate unless an individual has left instructions to the contrary. In Denmark, transplants were not available for many years because of the lack of agreement in defining 'brain death'; for some years patients needing heart, lung or liver transplants were sent to British, Dutch or German hospitals paid for from public funds. Parents in these countries were asked to donate organs from their brain dead child, whereas Danish parents were not asked on ethical grounds. Though WHO and the Council of Europe have both called for a prohibition of the trade in human organs and most European countries have made this trade illegal, Ireland and the Netherlands do not have any legislation on organ donation.

Research, particularly on pharmaceuticals, is often carried out in several centres in different countries. At present if pharmaceutical research is criticized on ethical or even methodological grounds in one country, it can be transferred to another European country where standards are not so high. The Second Helsinki Declaration on the ethics of medical research stated that experimental protocols should be submitted to a specially appointed independent committee for consideration, comment and guidance. Research ethics committees operate differently in each country, in terms of the number of committees, membership and the areas of research they cover; the involvement of users or lay people also varies. In some countries ethics committee members are mainly scientists, while others have equal numbers of scientists and lay members. In some countries lay members must be specialists in law, theology or philosophy. The problems for users and lay people on research ethics committees in the UK are outlined in Chapter 4.

Co-ordination of research ethics committees in different countries is required in order to ensure that multi-centre trials meet similar ethical standards, wherever they take place. The European Commission issued guidelines in 1990 which outlined the terms of reference for research ethics committees, but not the kind of national system that would enable co-ordination between European countries. Riis (1993) points out that it is important to create the types of national system that would make a European system possible.

Health rights

International charters of rights provide NGOs with a basis for campaigning in their own countries to improve services for their citizens. Some have no legal status, as those produced by consumer groups and WHO. While others, such as the UN Convention on the Rights of the Child, have a more formal status.

The European Region of the World Health Organization published the Declaration on the Promotion of Patients' Rights in Europe in 1994. The Declaration provides a framework for action, covering information, consent, confidentiality, privacy, care and treatment. It was developed after studies and surveys on the development of patients' rights throughout Europe and consultations with governments, professional and user bodies. Though countries varied in their legal frameworks, health care systems, economic conditions and social, cultural and ethical values, these studies showed that there were common approaches that could be adapted to the circumstances of each country (WHO, 1994). Comparative research identified two major concerns: that the 'imperatives of management, or profit, can be at odds with the well-being of patients' and that 'in the present context of budgetary restrictions and crisis in the welfare state . . . the most basic of rights could be under threat' (WHO, 1994: pviii, pxi).

The WHO Declaration provides guidelines only and these have not been put forward for formal adoption by member states. Several countries are looking at developing rights for patients, either through administrative systems with an ultimate recourse to law as in the UK or through legislation as in the Netherlands. Initiatives on patients' rights in the UK are discussed in Chapters 2 and 9. However, the WHO Declaration has been criticized (O'Keefe, 1996). The Declaration focuses on the individual user and the ethical problems that emerge as power shifts from clinicians to managers in health services. It was not set in a broad social context that looks at public health and health promotion, unlike WHO's Strategy for Europe. All the rights, except the right to care and treatment, are individual rights. The rights to care and treatment are social rights which specify that services should be equitable, appropriate to need, technically sound, culturally appropriate and humane. People from disadvantaged groups, such as from minority ethnic communities, often suffer from discrimination and difficulties in using services because of the way services are provided. These inequalities need to be addressed. Consumers International (1996) has produced a ten point Patients' Charter of basic rights that includes appropriate and accessible health care, freedom from discrimination, information and education, and informed consent about treatment. The charter was prepared for consumer groups to use as a basis for campaigning nationally.

Charters of patients' rights are not mandatory, but the UN Convention on the Rights of the Child is mandatory and was ratified by the UK government in 1991. The UN Charter established the rights of children and young people throughout the world, pointing to a child-centred approach to providing services to children and families, and the importance of social and economic conditions to help children live healthy lives. The UN Convention also specified the actions that governments needed to take to promote and guarantee these rights. The UK government has been criticized by a UN committee that monitors the observance of the Convention in each country (O'Keefe, 1996). It was particularly concerned about the lack of protection for the economic, social and cultural rights of children and the inequalities in the health status of children from different socio-economic groups and those belonging to ethnic minorities. High numbers of children were living in poverty. Gypsy and travelling children did not have access to basic services.

The principle that professionals must act in the best interests of the child is not embedded in UK law. As a result, for example, parents have the right to withdraw children from sex education in school; there is no right for the child to express an opinion. Though the Children Act 1989 is largely consistent with the child-centred approach of the Convention, it only applies to children defined as 'in need' and not to most services and facilities provided for children and young people. Nevertheless, by recognizing that children and young people have rights, not just their carers, the UN Convention has set a pattern for providing different sorts of services for children. Implementing the Convention should lead to changes in how health services are provided to children, in particular in areas of information, consent and access (BACCH, 1995).

Public health and health promotion

The EU started out as an economic community. Health, other than occupational health, has largely been seen as lying outside its remit. However, the EU is becoming more involved in health. Article 129 of the Maastricht Treaty on European Union states: 'Health protection requirements shall form a constituent part of the Community's other policies'. In 1996 the EU published the first annual report on public health in Europe, bringing together the relevant information on health from different directorates (EC, 1996). The European Parliament was one of the sources of pressure for extending the role of the EU in health and social affairs.

Other agencies, though their decisions are not mandatory on member states, can influence national developments. Initiatives which have had influence in the UK include WHO's global strategy of Health For All and related initiatives on Healthy Cities, Health Promoting Schools and UNICEF's Baby-Friendly Hospitals (Chapter 5). These initiatives provide ideas and support for professionals and NGOs to develop services in ways that promote health.

Health For All

The World Health Organization (WHO) was set up in 1948 as a specialized agency of the United Nations with primary responsibility for international health matters and public health. In the early days it concentrated on international programmes to eradicate particular diseases. This approach was very successful for smallpox, but did not work for malaria and measles. Furthermore, it became clear that health care could not be provided in developing countries along the same lines as in industrialized nations. In practical terms, there were not, and never could be, enough trained health staff to cover rural areas. Furthermore, health education was only effective if community leaders were involved and environmental improvements were made. Education about hygiene and avoiding infectious diseases could only work if communities could also obtain clean water and control malaria-carrying mosquitoes.

In response to these insights, WHO launched a global strategy in 1977 at Alma Ata with the target: *Health For All by the Year 2000*. It was based on six principles:

1　Equity in health both between groups in a country and between countries.
2　Primary health care as the focus of the health care system.
3　Health promotion, giving people a positive sense of health so that they can make full use of their physical, mental and emotional capacities.
4　Participation of local people in health services: *'health for all will be achieved by people themselves'*.
5　Multi-sectoral co-operation as the only way of effectively ensuring the prerequisites for health, promoting healthy policies and reducing risks in the physical, economic and social environment.
6　International co-operation: health problems transcend national frontiers. Pollution and trade in health-damaging products require international co-operation. (WHO, 1985)

With the Health For All (HFA) strategy, the WHO committed itself to an approach to health education that empowered local communities. It was committed to social justice and promoting equity within countries and also between rich and poor nations. Following the declaration at Alma Ata, WHO member states were urged to prepare national strategies, with targets for each region suited to its health priorities. With the HFA strategy the WHO moved from technical solutions for health problems to looking to political action to tackle inequalities in health. From the start, governments and professionals in the richer countries questioned whether this approach was relevant to them. They recognized that there were problems in health services in the 1970s: hospitals and acute medicine flourished at the expense of primary health care and little priority was given to prevention and public health. But it was not considered that a radical new framework was required – only a shift in attitudes and putting more resources into the less developed areas of health care. Furthermore, the principles of Health For All required a commitment at national level to social justice, the reduction of inequalities in health, and devolving power from central government to local level. These principles did not fit in with UK government policies in the 1980s.

In the UK the official HFA strategy focused on targets for specific diseases, tackling these through health education on individual lifestyles (such as smoking, alcohol and diet), immunization, and cancer screening (Chapter 3). HFA initiatives, such as Healthy Cities and Health Promoting Schools, have been taken up by NGOs and local authorities who were committed to the principles of equity, participation by local people and a holistic approach to health. Indeed recent trends have made some aspects of HFA appear more relevant to the UK – in particular by basing the health system in primary care rather than hospitals, and closer working between the NHS and local government. There is also support for more community participation and empowerment, which is integral to the WHO's strategy.

However, by moving into a political arena, WHO came into conflict with powerful commercial interests. For example, by promoting breast-feeding and taking a stand about the export and marketing of infant baby food to poor countries, it came into conflict with the manufacturers of baby food. When the WHO attempted to introduce a limited list of essential drugs, with the support of Health Action International, it came into conflict with the pharmaceutical industry. In the 1980s, the WHO began to focus again on programmes to control specific diseases. The focus on inequalities between the developed and less developed world was soon ignored and even the focus on inequalities within countries softened (O'Keefe, 1991). The WHO was also increasingly challenged and criticized for its cost, bureaucracy and lack of budgetary transparency (Walt, 1993).

The World Bank moved in to fill the policy vacuum left by the decline of the WHO. Set up after the Second World War to prevent another world war that might result from economic catastrophe, the World Bank offers long-term development assistance and is now a major funder of health and development projects worldwide. The World Bank has been criticized by NGOs for its narrow agenda that has led to an increase in inequalities between the richest and poorest countries (O'Keefe, 1995b). The World Bank has a different perspective on health and development from the WHO; the conflict between these approaches can be seen in maternity care. The WHO argued that poverty contributed to maternal deaths in developing countries; it promoted better training and support for traditional midwives. However, the World Bank promotes emergency obstetric care requiring anaesthesia, surgical equipment, oxygen and blood supplies, vacuum extraction equipment, medical personnel trained in doing Caesarean sections and efficient transportation (Novak, 1995).

Health promotion and trade

Health promotion can conflict with the interests of international trade and commerce. In the UK, taxation on cigarettes and alcohol is a way the government discourages people from drinking and smoking – as well as providing income for the Treasury. Taxes on cigarettes and alcohol are much lower in many European countries and so harmonization is likely to reduce the price of alcohol and cigarettes and increase consumption in the UK, which is likely to be opposed by health activists in the UK.

Though the EC is taking more and more account of the damage that trade policies can have on the health of its own citizens, it is not so concerned about the citizens of countries outside Europe, where the interests of European trade are put first. Drugs banned as unsafe in the USA and Europe continue to be marketed elsewhere and tobacco manufacturers have increased their marketing efforts in developing countries. An example is the sale and marketing of baby milk substitutes as a preferable option to breast milk. While health professionals firmly support breastfeeding as best for baby and mother, manufacturers want to market and promote their baby milk formulas. Since the 1970s there has been an international campaign against the marketing of baby milk substitutes. After complaints that the manufacturers, in particular Nestlé, marketed their products in a way that undermined breastfeeding, the International Code of Marketing Breast-milk Substitutes was adopted by WHO. In 1991 the EC agreed to ban the advertising and sale of some infant foods within but not outside Europe, overriding the views of the European Parliament. Lobbying by NGOs was successful in 1992 in getting the EC Directive controlling the export of baby foods to include more controls on labelling and details of composition.

However, there are many examples of breaches of the International Code by industry, both in Europe and in developing countries (IGBM, 1997). Baby Milk Action co-ordinates an international boycott of Nestlé's products and monitors and publicizes breaches of the Code. There are frequent attempts by the manufacturers' lobby to weaken regulations and enforcement. For example, since 1992 Nestlé has been buying up bottled water companies and, it is estimated, now controls over 10 per cent of the world market. In some countries the water is marketed as suitable for babies and for use in baby milk substitutes, using attractive pictures of healthy babies feeding from bottles (Baby Milk Action, 1997b).

Environmental protection

Pollution does not necessarily affect the polluter. One country can dispose of sewage and pollution into the sea or rivers, but it may be neighbouring countries that suffer damage. This is an area where the EC is increasingly concerned since the Single European Act (article 130) commits it: 'to preserve, protect and improve the quality of the environment'. Priorities include reducing pollution and nuisance from industry, the control of chemical substances and preparations, and the prevention of industrial accidents. The WHO and the EU have produced a Charter on the Environment which stresses the importance of considering the impact on health in policy formation at central level (WHO, 1990). It was a part of WHO's Health For All strategy and has been adopted by member governments. It included the principle that the polluter pays and supports the principle of sustainable development. Sustainable development aims to protect environments from degradation, pollution and overuse in order to meet the needs of people living now without compromising the ability of future generations to meet their own needs.

The principle of sustainable development is also the basis for Agenda 21. In 1992 at the 'Earth Summit' in Rio de Janeiro, Agenda 21 was signed by leaders from over one hundred and seventy countries, including the UK. It is an action plan to encourage people to develop more sustainable ways of living and to get involved in planning the future of their communities.

Agriculture

The European Union has been dominated by the Common Agricultural Policy (CAP) which guarantees a market to farmers for whatever they produce at guaranteed minimum prices. Sometimes health policy conflicts with agricultural policy. This conflict can be seen clearly in attitudes to tobacco smoking. Agricultural subsidies increased the number of tobacco producing countries in the EU from two to eight and the EU spends about £800m on subsidizing the production of tobacco that would probably not have been grown otherwise (Joosens and Raw, 1996). At the same time the EC funds anti-smoking campaigns and supports a ban on tobacco advertising.

Intensive agricultural production encouraged by CAP makes food cheap, but with undesirable long-term consequences for consumers and the environment. Pesticides and herbicides kill weeds and insects and help to keep the crop yields up but, as weeds and pests develop tolerance to chemicals, more and more are needed to have the same effect. There is increasing concern about the effects of pesticides on the health of both farmers and consumers, including fears that they may be causing cancers, asthma and damage to the immune system (Beaumont, 1993). There are different standards in different countries for the use of pesticides. In the UK, for example, the permitted levels are lower than in Germany.

Though EC agriculture policy is undergoing reform, there has been little discussion of the health implications of reform. There are ways that agricultural policy could improve health: for example, by making healthy foods such as fruit and vegetables cheaper and more readily available, and by decreasing the supply and raising the price of other products, such as sugars. The panic in Europe over the BSE crisis in Britain triggered renewed interest in public health issues in the EU. The implications of agricultural policies for health became clearer and public health issues across borders had to be taken seriously.

Nutrition and food safety

Regulation and harmonization of food and nutritional standards are needed in a free market to protect consumers. Infectious diseases can be spread by food distribution and there is increasing concern about the re-emergence of infectious diseases following the globalization of food distribution. New processes are also being developed that worry consumers, such as the use of hormones and antibiotics, and genetically modified food. These processes are not always covered by safety regulations because they are so new. For example, genetically engineered food – which involves changing the genetic structure of food – raises safety, environmental, religious and moral questions (Consumers International, 1997a). Labelling is also important since, without this, people with allergies or who do not want to consume genetically modified foods have no choice.

NGOs have had difficulties influencing food standards, while commercial interests are well represented on EC scientific committees through nutritionists with financial links with the food industry. Until 1996 members of the Scientific Committee for Food and ad hoc experts were not required to declare their interests. The only foods where content, as opposed to labelling, is regulated are those covered by the Foods for Particular Nutritional Uses Directive. The specialist rules produced under this Directive for infant formulas allow for up to 56 per cent of an infant formula to be sugars: sucrose was limited but not glucose. So manufacturers could advertise food that had very high sugar contents as being sucrose-free. By the time NGOs, such as the National Food Alliance and Action and Information on Sugars, found out about this they were told it was too late to change (AIS, 1991). Learning from this, NGOs attempted to get involved at an earlier stage, when standards for weaning foods – including baby drinks – were to be decided under this directive. This time the Department of Health gave the draft EC directive to UK NGOs for comment. The draft allowed for up to 15 per cent of baby drinks to be sugars – which is 50 per cent more than the sugar content of Coca-Cola. However, when consumer groups protested, they were informed once again that it was too late to change (AIS, 1993a). The draft was not really a draft: deals had already been done.

The World Trade Organization can now override decisions on food regulations made by the European Commission. The World Trade Organization was set up in 1995 under the General Agreement on Trade and Tariffs (GATT) to agree and regulate global trading standards. It, therefore, puts the interests of free trade above other interests. Consumers International has argued that it should develop a more transparent, accountable and participatory decision-making system (IOCU, 1994b). On nutrition and food safety the World Trade Organization is advised by the Codex Alimentarius Commission, which is a UN food standards agency set up in 1963 and run jointly by the Food and Agriculture Organization (FAO) and the WHO. Codex has a membership of over one hundred and thirty governments, and develops international food safety and quality standards to protect consumer health and, at the same time, facilitate trade.

With the establishment of the World Trade Organization, Codex is in a very powerful position to set world food standards. However, it has been criticized by consumer groups on the grounds that it has been dominated by the industry with little participation by consumers. In addition, it is not transparent in the way it works. Members are not required to declare any conflicts of interest in giving advice and some decisions are made by secret ballot. In 1993 the National Food Alliance surveyed participation in committees of Codex and concluded that public interest groups, as well as many national governments, were excluded whereas multinational organizations and industry federations were well represented (Avery et al., 1993). Twenty-six per cent of all participants on Codex committees represented industrial interests, while public interest organizations comprised only one per cent of total participation. On some committees, where consumer interest is particularly great, the industry representation was even higher. On one committee on food additives and contaminants, industry representation was 41 per cent and on nutrition and foods for special dietary uses it was 46 per cent. Consumers International (1997b) has been very concerned about the difficulties for consumers in participating in the Codex. In addition consumer organizations, unlike groups representing industry, do not have the funds to participate or be more strongly represented. This is particularly true of consumer organizations from developing countries.

Both the WHO and the FAO are concerned with nutritional standards, but their policies conflict. An example of the results of the different policies of the WHO and FAO can be seen in the International Conference on Nutrition held in 1992. This was a joint conference intended to promote better nutrition in both developed and developing countries. The nutritional standards supported by nutritionists in the UK and by the WHO emphasize the health problems caused by too much fat, sugar and salt in a diet. The FAO felt this approach to nutrition was inappropriate, since for people with too little to eat, any food was better than no food. An international expert advisory group of leading nutritionists was commissioned to prepare background scientific papers for the conference. The FAO insisted on the right to review and redraft the papers, which was done on its behalf by the chair of the nutrition committee of the International Life Sciences Institute. This Institute was founded in the 1970s by Coca-Cola and is a worldwide association of several hundred food multinationals, dominated by sweet food manufacturers. It funds research and publications that provide studies to use whenever there is public concern about the safety of their products. As a result the conference papers omitted all reference to sugars, which are particularly implicated in tooth decay and obesity. It is not perhaps surprising that the Declaration and Plan of Action that came from the conference did not mention sugar except as 'refined carbohydrates'. Ironically, the omission of sugar in the Declaration and Plan of Action has been used by the food industry in the UK to argue that the UK government is out of line in trying to reduce the sugar content in processed foods and in our diet (AIS, 1993b).

There is little leverage for consumers in this situation. Tim Lobstein of the Food Commission sums up the problems:

> As the regulations protecting the quality – including the environmental quality – of our food and our food production methods have been removed from local to national to international and then to global trading bodies immune to democratic processes, so we as individual purchasers and eaters of food must express our views through the last arena for action: the marketplace. We must learn to co-operate and co-ordinate our shopping practices, learn to combine our purchasing power to have some influence, and learn to express our concerns by demanding information and demanding change. (1996: 9)

Conclusions

It has been easier to describe the international events which affect us and are outside the control of a single national government than to illustrate how we, as users and citizens, can participate and influence them. Public interest groups need to work more closely together to influence these decisions. However, the problems for them mirror those faced at national level and are magnified: the difficulties of obtaining independent funding and information, the lack of transparency and accountability and the greater influence of rich commercial groups. Strengthening the voice of users and citizens in the European Union is essential to counterbalance the established powers of commercial interests.

International co-operation provides opportunities for users to learn from the experiences of other countries. As EU citizens, what people hear about the welfare systems in other countries may encourage them to press for equal advantages. Harmonization, which is increasing in pace, means that standards in some countries may be increased while in others they may be lowered. The question about harmonization, for consumers, is whether it works in favour of more consumer protection, public accountability and user involvement or less. For example, will harmonization of research ethics committees lead to more lay members or more scientists and professional members? With Sweden joining the EU, will this increase access to information or will it rather restrict freedom of information in Sweden?

Independent funding for NGOs to participate in international networks is required to strengthen the user lobby. The trend for NGOs to rely on funds from commercial companies may undermine the credibility of the user movement and this needs to be monitored. It may also lead to a split between the groups that see the major consumer issues to be in more regulation of commercial interests and those who are funded by them. In attempting to counterbalance other powerful and well-established lobbies, health interest groups need to make more alliances with other lobbies, in particular those concerned with the environment. Improvements in health care need to be sustainable and not result in future generations being at risk.

PART III
THE FUTURE

8

MYTHS ANCIENT AND MODERN

> Man must survive his dream which myth has both shaped and
> controlled. Society must cope with the irrational desires of its members.
> Ivan Illich, *Limits to Medicine – Medical Nemesis:*
> *the Expropriation of Health* (1975)

For most people, most of the time, health services are not important.
However, the existence of a National Health Service, available free to
any one who needs it, is of great importance. The NHS has been a symbol
that the government cares for the welfare of its citizens – in spite of the
harsh realities of unemployment and the financial struggles that many
people face. It is the only service where, as citizens, we undertake to share
according to need. In 1945 Winston Churchill promised Britain a health
service in which 'disease must be attacked in the poorest or in richest in
the same way as the fire brigade will give full assistance to the humble
cottage as readily as to the most important mansion' (quoted in Yates,
1995).

Since then there have been many changes and more are planned that
affect people's experiences of health and social care. There is commitment
at government level to involve users in these changes. However, there are
persistent and sometimes contradictory myths that dominate debates
about health policy, and justify and perpetuate the limited role that users
have. These need to be understood if users are to be able to contribute to
changing health and social care to meet their needs.

So far the relationships between health services and the public, as
patients and citizens, have been explored. In this chapter these relationships are put in the broader context of the trends that encourage more
involvement of users and those that go against it. Against this background,
some of the themes and myths that influence thinking about health policy
are discussed.

Ancient myths

Scientific certainty

Even the most sceptical of us believe, or want to believe, that a diagnosis means a treatment and treatment means a cure. The myth of medical and scientific certainty states that clinical diagnosis and treatment are based on rational scientific knowledge. However, in spite of our vast knowledge, there is little certainty in medicine and many common treatments are not scientifically proven to be effective. Even for routine conditions and with the most expert staff, it is not always possible to predict with certainty the outcome of treatment. Some people may not get better, though the prognosis was good. Others get better when they were expected to die.

One consequence of confidence in science can be unrealistic expectations among users and the public. Barham (1997) suggests that psychiatrists, by promising cures with new drugs for people with mental health problems, led people to expect too much. As a result of the failure or partial success of drug treatments for many people with mental health problems, there are increasing fears among the public of violent people who are mentally ill, encouraged by stories in the media. This has contributed to the perceived failure of community care policies and increased public pressure for more controls and segregation of people with mental health problems. The risk of violence for members of the public from mentally ill people may be very slight and there is no evidence that the risks are any greater than before, but the perception of the dangers influences public opinion – and ultimately public policy.

Putting your trust in scientific medicine can go badly wrong. Patients may be disillusioned if their expectations are not met, even if those expectations were unrealistic. Sharon Batt (1994) in her personal account, *Patient No More*, describes her voyage of discovery when she was diagnosed as having breast cancer. Like other women she had thought that breast cancer was a success story for modern medicine, but found this was not true. At the beginning of the twentieth century there was general pessimism about what could be done for people with cancer. Some doctors challenged this pessimism and allied with other professionals and philanthropists to see what could be done. In order to advance knowledge, they needed patients to ask for help and raise the profile of the disease in order to get funding. As clinicians and researchers have not been able to fulfil these hopes, it eventually led to a revolt and the breast cancer advocacy movement developed. Women felt that the belief that treatment could control breast cancer had put women at the mercy of commercial interests and the medical profession and removed them further from an understanding of themselves and their condition.

User groups have been formed to provide counter-information, such as the Association for Improvements in the Maternity Services, and newsletters, such as *What Doctors Don't Tell You*. Users have gained confidence from their awareness of the fallibility of the medical profession. Jean Robinson, describing a successful campaign against induction in labour in the 1970s, wrote:

> the induction disaster did wonders for consumer confidence. If doctors can make mistakes on that scale, our views on the way we gave birth were at least as good as theirs. We had learned, too, that knowledge is power. Once we had started reading the medical literature, we were not going to give up. (1995)

Awareness that health care can be a lottery led to interest in making clinical decisions on protocols based on evidence of effectiveness. Until recently, respect for the principle of clinical autonomy meant that doctors have not been required to base their clinical practice on evidence, follow treatment guidelines, or work as part of a team with nurses and other professionals – or even with each other. However, where there are such wide variations in diagnosis and recommended treatments between different clinicians and between different areas, nationally and internationally, there must be uncertainty about what is the best treatment. By the same token, there must also be much unnecessary treatment. This means that money could be saved if clinicians did not prescribe medicines or carry out treatments that were not clinically necessary – an attractive option for managers, economists and politicians.

Evidence-based medicine sensibly suggests that treatments should only be given where there is evidence that they actually work and improve health. This has enormous benefits for patients. It can provide information for them to make informed decisions and protect them from unnecessary or idiosyncratic treatment. It could also save money: if patients know the true odds and possible side effects, they may refuse some less effective treatments. Though evidence-based medicine is an important step forward, it faces some difficulties.

First, 'evidence' will be taken from published research, which is often of poor quality and about new drugs since so much is funded by the pharmaceutical industry (Chapter 4). Much research looks only at symptoms, not causes, and at the short-term effects on patients. Much less research is undertaken on the long-term impact on patients and their quality of life, or on non-drug alternatives which may cost less than medicines.

Secondly, there are pressures against evidence-based medicine from the public, professionals and the private sector. If doctors can 'do something', even if the evidence is against treatment, some doctors may be prepared to do it – if the money is available and patients and carers want it. A situation could arise where the NHS restricts the treatments available based on what makes medical sense, while the private sector provides treatment which is not medically justified. For example, Child 'B', Jaymee Bowen, first contracted lymphoma with leukaemia when she was six years old. She was given a bone marrow transplant but developed myeloid leukaemia. The clinicians in charge, both at Addenbrooke's and the Royal Marsden Hospitals, decided that a further bone marrow transplant was unlikely to be successful when she was ten. Her father took the health authority to court in 1995, but the court ruled that the decision was up to the health authority. The treatment would have cost £75 000, and media publicity focused on the savings that the health authority was making by refusing further treatment. Money was provided by an anonymous donor and Jaymee received treatment in a private hospital. This was not a bone marrow transplant but a new treatment, donor lymphocyte infusion, that had not been tried on a child before. It was also, incidentally, carried out by a doctor without paediatric training or experience of children with this condition. Jaymee Bowen died in May 1996 after a year of remission (New, 1996).

The public may be reluctant to accept a realistic but more pessimistic view of what doctors can achieve. When faced with death, especially of a child or young person, treatments that provide hope – whatever the risks and costs – often seem preferable to the alternatives that do not offer hope. Learning to live with cancer or a heart condition is learning to live with uncertainty. This may be hard to accept, even if there is no evidence that treatment will make a difference to the length of life and may even reduce the quality of the time remaining. Some women from families with a history of breast cancer choose to have double mastectomies rather than wait to see if they are going to develop cancer. The treatment they choose is a more drastic one than the treatment given to women who actually have cancer.

While evidence-based medicine looks at specific interventions, public health professionals are adopting the idea of evidence-based health policies. This aims at devising policies that are most likely to benefit the health of communities, which moves away from the focus on specific interventions and the medical model to look at 'health gain'. The evidence-base for specific interventions constantly changes as new drugs are produced and new research is published. The evidence for interventions that improve public health is more stable and provides a broader base for health planning.

Medical progress

Along with the myth of scientific certainty goes the myth of progress in medicine. This states that science can and will conquer disease – given sufficient time and resources – and is continually pushing back the frontiers of disease and pain. Though there have been some amazing medical breakthroughs, like antibiotics in the 1940s, they are not as common or as dramatic as the media or researchers would have us believe. Medicine has taken the credit for dramatic improvements in health caused by the reduction in diseases such as measles, whooping cough and TB. These are often assumed to be due to the introduction of antibiotics, sulphonamide drugs for TB and immunization programmes. These improvements were, however, a success story for the nineteenth-century public health movement. They were brought about by improvements in social and environmental conditions – clean water, sanitation, better working conditions, housing and nutrition. The development of antibiotics and vaccines assisted in the decline that was already well advanced (DHSS, 1976).

The history of medicine has had many false starts and breakthroughs that led nowhere. Some now seem bizarre, but they were based on the best intentions and the best knowledge at the time. As Charles Medewar of Social Audit puts it:

> The history of medicine is rarely taught in medical schools. The real reason may be that so much of it is an 'embarrassment', but the conventional wisdom is that medicine has advanced so far since the early days that there would be little point in looking back. The prevailing view in medicine is always that great strides have been made, and that patients have never had it so good. (1992: 12)

In spite of the resources and publicity given to cancer research, progress has been limited. Knowledge has increased enormously, but this does not always lead to effective treatment or cures. As long ago as 1972, Lord Zuckerman published a report on cancer research. He concluded that research had failed to produce results – even though there was no shortage of funds, facilities or scientists hard at work. The problem was a shortage of ideas. Since then radiotherapy, surgery and chemotherapy have been refined and improved but, except for specific cancers, the results have not been substantial. A report published in 1997 in the USA concluded that:

> The war against cancer is far from over. Observed changes in mortality due to cancer primarily reflect changing incidence or early detection. The effect of new treatments for cancer on mortality has been largely disappointing. The most promising approach to the control of cancer is a national commitment to prevention with a concomitant rebalancing of the focus and funding of research. (Bailar and Gornik, 1997)

Lesley Doyal and Samuel Epstein have argued that the problem of the rise in cancers may not be so much scientific as political and economic. Causes that lie in the individual are exaggerated at the expense of researching hazards that lie in the environment (Doyal et al., 1983).

Medical progress is not straightforward and treatment is not always beneficial. Sometimes treatment can cause more problems for patients than the original illness. There is also the increasing problem of iatrogenic diseases – that is, illnesses that have been caused by sound and professionally recommended treatment. In 1975 in *Medical Nemesis*, Ivan Illich made a powerful case for the extent of iatrogenic diseases and the impact they had on health. Hospitals are dangerous places where infections or bed sores are picked up. About one in ten patients in hospital at any one time has an infection picked up while there. One in five patients in intensive care are estimated to have an infection acquired since they were admitted (OHE, 1997).

Perhaps the most chilling example of iatrogenesis in drugs is the long-term effects of some drugs for mental illness. In the 1950s and 1960s neuroleptic drugs were introduced for schizophrenia. It is now estimated that up to a half of people who take these drugs long-term develop tardive dyskinesia, a disease that causes brain damage and uncontrollable twitches and spasms for which there is no known treatment. The drug company Roche Laboratories estimated in 1980 that 150 million people worldwide were receiving neuroleptics at that time, which means that millions of people worldwide must be suffering from brain damage induced by these drugs (Breggin, 1993).

The media also encourage optimism with 'good news' stories about magic bullets to kill cancers and research breakthroughs. Good press coverage of research is needed in order to maintain confidence in the expertise of doctors and to ensure that funding is available for research, but it can also give a selective and over-optimistic view of scientific progress (Karpf, 1988). Scientific research is generally a hard grind as knowledge is built up slowly, with few discoveries about which researchers can shout 'eureka'. In contrast, in the media world, certainties and extremes of good or bad news make the headlines. Some clinicians have pointed out the difficulties that these 'good news' stories create for them. People come to them armed with magazine or newspaper articles and find it difficult to accept that the new treatment is not available and will not be available for many years, if at all. The myth of medical progress is maintained because we want to believe; and because there are profits to be made from new drugs and techniques.

There are some disconcerting reasons why an increase in knowledge does not always lead to a long-term improvement in health. This is because, in biology, all progress is relative (Ridley, 1994). This concept is called the 'Red Queen'. In *Alice in Wonderland*, the Red Queen has to keep running in order to stay in the same place, since the landscape moves with her. If she wants to travel to another place, she has to run twice as fast. The more progress you appear to make, the more the world moves with you and the less actual progress you make. For two generations, infectious diseases and diseases caused by parasites and bacteria seemed to be under control; they could be prevented by immunization but, even if they developed, they could be treated easily. However, as soon as we have learnt to kill these bugs, they have adapted and learnt to overcome or circumvent medical treatments. Many infectious diseases, like TB and malaria, are making a comeback and new ones are also emerging (Garrett, 1994). Antibiotics are no longer as effective and there are already 'superbugs' that resist them. The landscape of illness is keeping up with us and we have to make greater and greater efforts to keep ahead. The phenomenon of the Red Queen means that it is important to keep investing in research in order to stay still.

A new perspective on disease is also provided by evolutionary medicine. This suggests that many aspects of what we think of as disease are actually the side effects of benefits that have evolved over time (Nesse and Williams, 1995). For example, for people living in Northern countries there is a benefit in having a lighter skin which is better able to synthesize Vitamin D when exposed to sunlight and this can prevent rickets. For people living in places with little sunlight, a pale skin is therefore an advantage. The problems come when light skinned people go and live in sunny areas such as Australia or expose their bodies to intensive sun on holidays. They may get melanomas, a potentially fatal skin cancer which has increased greatly in recent years. Sickle cell disorders are caused by genes that are also useful. The gene that causes sickle cell anaemia is most common in people from areas where there is malaria. Someone who carries the gene is less likely to get malaria in early childhood. Only when you inherit the gene from both parents, do you get sickle cell anaemia.

Heroic medicine

It was recognized in the 1970s that some parts of the country had poorer health care than others, and that some services were inadequate and undeveloped. These 'Cinderella' services included community services, and services for the elderly and people with disabilities, mental health problems and learning difficulties. Improving them was seen to be a matter of redistributing resources from over-bedded acute hospitals in London to poorer areas and to these Cinderella services. However, these attempts to shift resources within the health service failed. This was mainly because of the power of the medical profession and the acute hospitals which preferred to see health care in terms of heroic interventions rather than caring for people with chronic conditions.

According to the myth of heroic medicine, diseases are short acute episodes that need quick interventions, and the priority of medicine and health care is to battle against disease with aggressive interventions. Both doctors and patients believe in the potential value of interventions and the importance of trying everything, against all the odds and even the evidence. Death comes to be seen as a failure of medicine. In reality, most illnesses are long-term or disabling conditions that people live with. Heart disease, many cancers and all hip replacements are chronic conditions and effective treatment involves helping people to learn to live with the condition. You also have to learn to live with the possibility that you will have another heart attack, the cancer will return or your hip will deteriorate. By focusing on cure and repair, learning to live with disability, pain or chronic illness becomes second best.

There are several implications of the belief in heroic medicine for health services. First, as medicine becomes more complex and depends more on high technology, there is more specialization. There are over forty recognized clinical specialties, each concentrating on particular parts of the body or particular functions, with little co-ordination between specialists. Dividing individuals into constituent parts makes it difficult to look at them as whole people. It encourages clinicians to be detached from and not value the subjective experiences of patients.

Secondly, this belief leads us to concentrate on some causes of ill health but ignore others. It looks for the causes of disease in bacteria or viruses – alien intruders to be expelled or controlled. It looks for causes in the genes that are inherited from parents, that make people susceptible to heart disease or particular cancers; it looks for causes in the way people choose to live – too much drinking, smoking or stress. It does not look for causes of disease in the environment and cannot explain the vast inequalities in health between people in different socio-economic and ethnic groups.

Thirdly, in the past the belief in heroic medicine affected the way that health services were organized and how resources were spent on health care. It justified spending money on hospital and specialist services rather than on primary care, community services or continuing care. The belief in heroic medicine also justified research into new cures and treatment, often looking at the short-term results of interventions rather than at what happens to people who have treatment over a longer period or how people cope with living with the side effects of drugs or the results of surgery.

We want the best health care for ourselves and our families. Sometimes this may mean heroic interventions, but always giving priority to new technologies and drugs tends to mean that other services suffer. Money is found to fund new expensive drugs for a few people, while basic standards which affect the lives of many more people deteriorate.

Modern myths

Infinite demand and rationing

In the 1980s there was a perception that the costs of health care were out of control and that we, as a society, could not afford to pay for modern health care. Similar financial crises were faced by countries all over the world, whether health services were based on insurance schemes or funded by general taxation. As the costs of health care escalated, the priority for managers was to contain these costs which meant that they had to have more control over what doctors did. The *Griffiths Report* of 1983 criticized the NHS for lack of direction and leadership and recommended that general managers be introduced throughout the NHS (DHSS, 1983). Managers acquired more power and status as new organizational structures were introduced.

A new myth developed as a result of concern about the escalating costs of health care: the myth that demand for health care is infinite, but resources are finite. The task of managers was to curb the demand for health care and control patients' expectations. The NHS was planned on assumptions current in the 1930s that there was a limited amount of morbidity which, if tackled, would lead to less sickness and lower health service costs in the long term. These assumptions now seem hopelessly naive.

However, the demand for much health care is finite. Only a limited number of people need hip replacements or hernia repairs. In addition, the amount of resources that are available to spend on health care is a political decision and a question of priorities. Any government could decide to put up taxes or divert money from defence or road building to health care. Compared to other European countries, the costs of health care in the UK are low and reports from the Institute for Public Policy Research maintained that the NHS could cope with increased demands (Wordsworth et al., 1996). The House of Commons Select Committee also reported in 1996 that long-term care for elderly people could be afforded from taxation (House of Commons Select Committee, 1996).

The founders of the NHS did not anticipate how 'demand' could be created and how the definitions of sickness and health would be redefined.

HOW DEMAND IS CREATED   There are many reasons for increased demand. First, some of the increased demand is due to medical advances. Many people can be treated with drugs or other treatments, when before they would have been told that nothing could be done. Secondly, new diseases, such as AIDS, are emerging and the incidence of others such as asthma is rising. Others, such as TB and malaria, are making comebacks and becoming resistant to established drugs. At the same time there has been a rise in diseases associated with poverty, unemployment, and living and working in an unhealthy environment. Thirdly, people are living longer, though often in poor health, and need care and treatment in old age. Over forty per cent of health service resources are spent on treating people over 65. Finally, people have higher and higher expectations of the health service, in particular they want more information, more choice and more time for consultations.

Demand can be created by offering treatments, that are considered to be effective, to more people. Some interventions which are now considered to be given unnecessarily developed in this way, including hysterectomies, Caesarean sections, D&Cs, grommets and tonsillectomies. When angioplasty was first developed, it was assumed that it would replace coronary artery bypass grafts. However, both techniques have increased and the criteria for carrying out bypass operations and angioplasty have been lowered to include people with heart conditions without symptoms (Graboys et al., 1992). Some conditions, previously seen as normal, may be reclassified or treated as if they are diseases: pregnancy, the menopause, weight or height.

Often 'demand' is created by clinicians motivated by altruism, optimism and scientific curiosity to try out new techniques and drugs. Doctors can now do a lot more than even a few years ago. And the more they can do, the more they want to do and are expected to do. New drugs, such as beta interferon and Viagra, create new demands and incur new costs. For example, beta interferon is a drug for the relapsing remitting form of multiple sclerosis, which seems to help reduce the symptoms though does not affect the progression of the disease. The drug costs about £10 000 a year per patient and if all patients who might benefit were treated, the total cost could be as much as ten per cent of the NHS drugs bill (Whalley and Barton, 1995).

Research into genes is opening major new areas. It has been predicted that by the year 2010 almost 30 per cent of all health care expenses in Western countries will stem from gene therapy (NCC, 1995).

The public also may demand drugs or services. Both cervical and breast cancer screening programmes were introduced because of lobbying by professionals and women, but they have not yet delivered the expected benefits (Chapter 3). Once programmes are set up, there is too much investment and too many expectations among the public to close them down. Screening creates a demand for testing and diagnosis but also provides the opportunities to 'treat' whatever illness or 'imbalance' is found. Inevitably some people will receive treatment that they do not need, especially if the provider is paid for each treatment that is given.

Commercial interests are in the business of creating demand so that they can provide products and services to meet it. Drug companies are now selling their products directly to the public, even advertising them on television. In this way they create awareness of the possible benefits of their products and create new markets. Based on information provided by commercial organizations and professionals, users may campaign for new drugs to be available and rushed through the licensing procedures. Sometimes these drugs have not been adequately tested or their benefits proven. Pressures from users can lead to a serious tension between public demand and effectiveness, undermining rational planning of health and social services and increasing costs.

Broadening health care from a unified public system to a diverse market of competing providers has encouraged the development of a profitable health market. Private services are not concerned with public health or the care of people with chronic conditions. As a result the growth in the private health care market is not likely to lead to the improved health status of the population as a whole. This has been the experience in the USA, which spends far more on health care in absolute dollar terms and relative to their gross domestic product than anywhere else in the world. Expenditure was 14 per cent in 1992, compared to 7.1 per cent in the UK and a mean for OECD countries of 8.4 per cent. Of this the public share of total spending on health in the USA was 45.7 per cent, compared to an OECD mean of 74.7 per cent and in the UK 84.4 per cent (OECD, 1995).

Even with this expenditure, one in seven Americans is not covered by health insurance and many others are faced with the risk of losing insurance cover if they become unemployed. The USA also has the poorest results in terms of life expectancy, infant mortality and access to care for its citizens, as well as the lowest value for money in terms of the costs, the number of professional visits, consultations and admissions to hospital compared to other Western countries (Schieber and Pouiller, 1990).

RATIONING AND CONTROLLING DEMAND   If demand, however it is created, is escalating, the question is how to control it. There is nothing new about 'rationing'. There was in the 1960s and 1970s, and still is, a lack of investment in community services, mental health services and services for people with learning difficulties. Rationing was achieved by not investing funds in developing services or research, and by giving staff low pay, low status and poor training.

Rationing debates tend to assume that medicine is always good; the question is how to spread it around. Waiting lists have been a long-established way of managing demand in a health service with free access. People in urgent need of treatment receive it immediately, while those in less urgent need have to wait. Waiting lists became a major political issue following the Patient's Charter in 1991 and this led to a perception that waiting for treatment, whether urgent or not, was unacceptable. However, waiting lists may be a fairer way of managing demand than many others, as long as they take account of the deterioration, pain and disability of those waiting. In contrast, costs in the USA are contained by allowing a large number of the population to be uninsured, so they do not receive health care. There are increasing problems in the USA as more and more people are being refused insurance because they have pre-existing conditions and are 'too high a risk' for insurers to take on.

If waiting lists are not acceptable, other ways of controlling demand have to be found. There are a number of different approaches to 'rationing'. People may be refused treatment perhaps because of their age or lifestyle. Some treatments may be excluded because they are not considered effective or important, such as IVF or gender reassignment. People may also be deterred from using services by making them difficult to access or by introducing charges. There are many practical and ethical difficulties in discussions about 'rationing'; Mullen (1995) has pointed out that 'rationing' may not be necessary and that there may be alternatives.

Nevertheless, debates about rationing cause public anxiety. People are no longer confident that services will be there when they need them. These anxieties can persuade employers and individuals to take out private health insurance and use private health services. This enables publicly funded services to concentrate on those who cannot afford to pay and saves money for them in the short term. However, this will lead to some people receiving too much treatment for their own health and some too little. Furthermore, people who are privately insured are less likely to support greater NHS spending than those who are not (Besley et al., 1996). If cuts in services lead to more people taking out private health insurance, this could lead to a downward spiral and may result in pressure for lower spending. This could result in the publicly funded health services becoming a safety net – like Medicaid in the USA – with the principle of equity lost.

Rationing, whether implicit or explicit, has always existed. Decisions on what services to provide and what to 'ration' need to be based on evidence of effectiveness and on information about who is likely to benefit. Rationing decisions in the UK are left to local health authorities – because this way politicians avoid controversy and the blame for unpopular decisions that result from lack of resources. However, this may increase inequalities between different areas. Rationing needs to be undertaken as part of developing a comprehensive health care system, based on looking at the feasibility of satisfying demand and at the health needs of the community (Williams and Frankel, 1993).

The patient as consumer

Alongside the myth of infinite demand has developed the myth that the patient is a consumer. By exercising choice, consumers can help to manage the health care market and make it more consumer-centred – or so runs the theory of the market. Managers in the 1980s attempted to 'satisfy' their consumers or customers, but in time consumers began to demand to be satisfied – a different power relationship altogether. Patients, armed with the Patient's Charter, were encouraged to demand their rights as consumers and so influence how services were provided for them. For professionals these changes have brought additional stresses. Later there was a backlash and in 1997 the Labour Government announced that the Patient's Charter would be replaced by a new NHS Charter that gave patients responsibilities and not simply rights.

Consumers are assumed to know their own best interests and what they want and so the balance of power shifts back to them from professionals. Nevertheless, the consumer model does not fit well into health care. In public services it is difficult even to define who the consumer is. Is the consumer the patient or the carer? The parent or the child? Almost thirty years ago Richard Titmuss summarized the difficulties (1969: 67): medical care is uncertain and unpredictable; many consumers do not desire it, do not know they need it, and cannot know in advance what it would cost them. They cannot learn from experience. They must rely on the supplier to tell them if they have been well served, and cannot return the service to the seller or have it repaired. Medical services are not advertised as other goods and the producer discourages comparisons. Once the purchase is made, consumers cannot change their minds in mid-treatment. Medical producers have the power to select their consumers, if need be, by the intervention of the police: the producers can even sell forcible internment and asylums.

Consumers need unbiased information with which to make choices about services and treatment and who should provide them. This requires open access to information about the effectiveness and outcome of treatments and the performance, qualifications and experience of providers. However, those providing services have incentives to keep this information from consumers or to manipulate the information to influence people to use their consumer power in particular ways.

By contrast to the UK, in France patients have consumer choice. The French health care system is complex, based on universal health insurance with independent and public providers. The principles, laid down in the 1920s, gave patients the right to choose their doctor, and doctors have the freedom to prescribe and practice where they wish. Patients can refer themselves directly to specialist services without first going to a GP and they can see whichever doctor they want. People in France appreciate the power they have. A study of ten countries showed high levels of satisfaction in France where 41 per cent thought the system worked pretty well and only minor changes were needed (compared to 27 per cent in the UK). In France, 52 per cent thought that fundamental changes were needed or the system completely rebuilt, compared to 69 per cent in the UK. In general, satisfaction was related to the amount of money spent (apart from in the USA), presumably because there was less waiting, staff were less stressed and there were better facilities (Blendon et al., 1990). However, a report from the Organisation for Economic Co-operation and Development (OECD) pointed out that there are problems where consumers have choice and providers have autonomy as they do in France. Patients are not in a position to question the advice of doctors and they have no reason to restrain their demands for care. As a result intervention rates and costs are higher and long-term care is poor. The OECD (1992) suggests that a better system would give 'consumer' choice to the insurer rather than the patient since the insurer takes account of costs and quality to engender competition through the system. This is in fact the situation in the NHS, where consumer power in the health market lies with the purchaser of services rather than with users. Purchasers – health authorities, GPs and insurance companies – have choice and are able to influence the nature and quality of services provided.

The focus on consumerism and the individual has distracted us from recognizing the importance of democratic accountability and collective public involvement. Patients and the public were first given a role in the 1974 NHS reorganization when it was recognized that 'lay' people, represented by community health councils, could be an important counterbalance to professional power. Then the focus moved away from community and collective approaches to participation towards a focus on the individual patient as consumer. Choice and personal freedom are important values but they may come into conflict with equity. In the

USA the health care system developed from the values of personal responsibility, freedom of choice and pluralism. In the UK and Europe the health care system developed from values of achieving a healthy population and equality of access to services for everyone. A balance between individual rights and equity, and collective rights is complex but important to achieve.

The patient as partner

There is now a new myth – that patients can be partners with government, professionals and pharmaceutical companies. Department of Health set up a Patient Empowerment Unit in 1991 to strengthen the relative position of users in health care. In 1996 the NHS Executive launched the idea of patient partnerships as the basis for a collaborative strategy, replacing the earlier focus on patient empowerment, which was more threatening and antagonistic to professionals (NHSE, 1996b). The Doctor Patient Partnership is a BMA and the Department of Health initiative to inform people how to use health services more responsibly. Partners for Better Health Care is a pharmaceutical company initiative which funds meetings and newsletters for patients groups.

However, partnerships require the benefits and the risks of joint ventures to be shared. Though users have some shared concerns with professionals and pharmaceutical companies, they also have very different interests which may conflict with the interests of the other 'partners'. Furthermore the 'risks' they take are different from those taken by professionals or pharmaceutical companies. Patients have much more to win and much more to lose: the type of health care they receive may be a matter of life or death.

Partnership is an attractive concept that builds on common interests, but raises problems. The first problem may be that if people believe in partnerships they may overlook the genuine conflicts within health policy. Even the Department of Health itself has a conflict of interest in that it aims to promote the pharmaceutical industries and at the same time ensure that the NHS has access to safe, effective and affordable medicines. The corporate public relations (PR) of transnational companies have been very successful in promoting a favourable business climate – 'engineering consent' (Richter, 1998). If people fail to recognize different interests, or deny conflicts exist or are justified, democratic debate is stifled. If conflict and conflicts of interests are not recognized for what they are, the interests of the more powerful will inevitably win.

The second problem is the inequality between users and other partners in their access to resources and decision making. In fact voluntary groups often rely on funding from government, professional and commercial interests to survive at all. This means that users may be funded to undertake activities that also benefit other 'partners', whether fundraising for research or for diagnostic equipment for a clinical specialty, or helping to promote particular drugs or treatments. For example, a pharmaceutical company funds a scheme to use people with arthritis who are trained as patient partners to train professionals in the diagnosis and management of arthritis. This scheme values the views and experiences of patients, but may also turn the patient partners into effective sales representatives for the company. Furthermore, it may lead to divisions within the user movement between those that work in 'partnership' and those who do not.

Accepting funding from other 'partners' enables voluntary groups to do good things that they could not otherwise do, but may also provide – at the very least – effective PR for commercial or professional interests and may also do much more in promoting their causes. Groups that do not undertake activities that support other 'partners', or who are suspicious of the motives of the other partners, are likely to be dismissed as negative and unhelpful and may be excluded from dialogue. Their views will not be heard.

The perfectibility of health

Now that there is less optimism about medical progress and less trust in the infallibility of doctors, people have become less compliant and ask more questions. They want, and are encouraged, to take a more active role in their health care and in promoting their own health – through a healthy lifestyle, buying health enhancing products, screening and alternative or complementary therapies. This has led to the myth of the perfectibility of health. Illness is no longer something that just happens to us; we can determine our own health, if we are prepared to work for it. We may feel alright but we could feel better – with more exercise, taking vitamins or using alternative practitioners.

This has enormous implications for health policy, as discussed in Chapter 3. The boundaries of health and ill-health can be shifted, creating new demands and new markets for health care and products – including alternative and complementary therapies. Screening for high or low blood pressure will produce an enormous number of extra people considered to require treatment. Again, being short, which may be genetically determined, may be seen as a disability, especially in boys. A child may be given growth hormones so that they can be nearer the 'normal' height. Similarly, the menopause, instead of being a natural stage in a woman's life, is now often described as an abnormal condition. Hormone replacement therapy is promoted, not just for women who have problems, but for all women.

Mental illness is also an area where the boundaries between health and illness are constantly changing. Medical treatment for mental illness only developed in this century, with ECT, psychosurgery and drugs. As the old asylums closed, there was an increase in the awareness of mental health problems in the community. Psychiatrists were able to offer drugs and so extended their interests from people in hospital to people in the community. Gradually the term mental illness has been replaced by mental health. This, at first glance, seems positive and less stigmatizing but also has implications for the boundaries of mental health services. Tranquillizers became 'mother's little helper' and by the mid 1970s only one tranquillizer prescription in eight was for a recognized psychiatric disorder. Drugs, like Prozac, are seen as a way of enhancing performance rather than dealing with illness as such.

The belief in the perfectibility of health is implicit in the World Health Organization's definition of health as a state of complete physical, mental and social well-being. This seems an aspiration that no one can achieve for more than an hour, or day, at a time. The belief that illness is not something to be accepted and lived with has implications for everyone. It can lead people to feel anxious and worried about illnesses they may never have and become more dependent on 'experts' and make more demands on health services.

Conclusions

Professor Julian Le Grand (1997) suggests that health policy in the past, and in the present, has been based on incorrect assumptions about how people behave. Health policy was based on the assumption that people who financed, operated and used the welfare state were public spirited altruists (that is, knights) and the passive recipients of state largess (patients and clients) were pawns. With the internal market this view changed to see both providers and recipients of services as, in one way or the other, self-interested (that is, knaves). Both these views are incorrect but inhibit rational planning of health services. There has been a further shift. As managers, accountants and economists replaced clinicians in dominating health policy, the medical profession has been recast as altruistic knights, defending the rights of the individual patient and ethical standards against managers and accountants who are now the knaves.

These assumptions continue in some of the myths surrounding health care. The myths justify the high status of experts, whether clinicians, managers or auditors, and limit the part that outsiders can play in making choices for themselves as patients or questioning policies as citizens. Even the myth of the patient as consumer does not necessarily give users more power. Effective consumerism requires open access to information and to redress, but the information and choices available to users are limited by professional and other interests. The focus on individual rights also means that there is less interest in increasing public accountability or democracy in health services.

Furthermore, these myths encourage us to equate health with health care – which creates new markets and a demand for more health care and more 'cures'. While we may consume health care, this may not give us health. In fact, there is a point where more health care endangers health and people may receive unnecessary interventions or experience side effects of treatments. These myths all divert attention away from inequalities in health among different groups in the community that have increased since the 1980s. Reducing poverty and unemployment, providing better housing or improving the environment are likely to achieve better health for the nation than will health care.

There is agreement that health care is in crisis, but there is no consensus about what is to be done. Tackling the problems that are faced by all health services requires users and citizens to be in the centre of decision making, whether about their own bodies, the way that services are organized and managed or public policies that affect health and welfare. How this might be achieved is discussed in the final chapter.

9

TAKING OVER

The reasonable man adapts himself to the world; the unreasonable man
persists in trying to adapt the world to himself. Therefore all progress
depends on the unreasonable man.

George Bernard Shaw *Man and Superman* (1903)

There is no consensus about how health services should be organized or
funded. Should taxation be increased, insurance schemes set up as in
other European countries or should services provided by the NHS be
restricted? The 'visions' that abound are often exercises in thinking the
'unthinkable' and moving away from consensus, rather than building
on it. Gradually the unthinkable becomes acceptable. The lack of shared
values in health policy results in a worried and disgruntled public, low
morale among staff, and indecision in health service management. This
inevitably affects the quality of services.

Since the nineteenth century the medical profession has dominated
health care. This has led to a service where experts have acted in the best
interests of their patients: a health service that has mixed excellence
in some acute specialties with appalling standards of care in less popular
areas, such as mental health. Not only were resources spread unfairly
between specialties and between geographical areas, but costs to the state
escalated.

So managers took over the leadership of the health service in the 1980s,
again acting in the 'best interests' of customers or consumers. This led,
in turn, to a health service driven by the 'market', with patients acting
as consumers to help bring about change. This failed to contain costs.
It increased inequalities and alienated the public who did not like the
language of business applied to a popular public service. The focus then
changed to a 'primary care-led' health service.

The ten-year programme outlined in the White Paper, *The New NHS –
Modern, Dependable,* provides a commitment to involving users. The test
of its effectiveness may be in how the position of users and the public
is strengthened as the programme unfolds. This chapter explores the
changes that are required to provide a health policy and health service
based on the experiences and views of users.

Health promoting society

The quality of our lives and mental health depends to a large extent on income, employment, housing, the pleasantness of the environment and being able to walk safely in the street. The question is, how much are people prepared to contribute financially in tax? How far are the profits and economic benefits that commercial companies generate given priority over health? How seriously are environmental pollution, food safety, and safety in the workplace taken?

The answers to these questions affect the sort of society we live in. In the UK, expenditure on health services is lower than most other European countries and food is cheaper. Opinion polls suggest people would be prepared to pay more taxes for better services. In spite of this it is accepted 'wisdom' that voters do not mean it and that any political party who called this bluff and offered better public services or consumer protection in exchange for higher taxes would be defeated in an election. This may be true, but it is arrogant to assume it without stronger evidence.

Health needs to be put before health care. An informed debate requires a national health strategy where health interests are taken into account in decisions by all government departments. It must also be recognized that health care and health promotion are big industries and that there are vested commercial and professional interests involved. A national public health strategy may help to reduce inequalities in health. Richard Wilkinson (1996) has shown that large differences in income between the richest and poorest in a society reduce social cohesion in that society. Furthermore, in modern economies, narrower income differences are associated with faster not slower economic growth. Reducing inequalities requires a debate about social and substantive rights that relate to the obligations that society has: obligations to make reasonable provision for health care for the population and to ensure equal access to health care for all those living in a country and the elimination of discrimination – whether on financial, geographical, ethnic, cultural, social or psychological grounds.

Public accountability and participation

The NHS is run by people who have been selected, not elected. Selection relies on patronage and inevitably favours people who are established and who are deemed to be 'experts'. In consequence the health service has little democratic accountability, and secrecy and lack of scrutiny has enabled vested interests to influence decisions behind the scenes. Democratic accountability, as well as integrated health and social care, could be achieved if local government became responsible for commissioning health and social care and took the lead in public health. A report from the Institute for Public Policy Research suggests that local authorities could become 'commissioners for health', covering medical services, long-term care, and preventive strategies as well as environmental health, social services, education and housing (Harrison et al., 1991). The management of hospitals and health services could remain, separately, within the Department of Health.

In order to ensure accountability and encourage participation, openness in the way decisions are made and access to information are essential. A Freedom of Information Act should enable the influence of different interest groups to be more easily identified, in particular the links that are often present between commercial interests, professionals and politicians. Making discussions more open will enable people to understand better, not only the nature of health and disease, but also the complexity of issues – for example, those around 'rationing' or controlling new drugs and technologies.

In addition to elected representatives and more open decision making, there need to be structures to enable people to participate in and contribute to local, national and international debates. The 'community' is made up of many different groups with different concerns, needs and priorities that often conflict. Arrangements for consultation and participation need to cover all local services that affect people's lives and cannot easily be separated: health care, social care, the environment, housing and community safety. A community-based body, building on experiences of CHCs, could be established to assist people to participate in local health and local authority services and help them make better use of them. It could co-ordinate local community forums that advise on commissioning and monitor local services.

Achieving wider participation involves a long-term investment of resources to encourage and support people, and give them the confidence and information to participate in an informed way. This needs to start with young people and in schools. Just as important, managers and staff need training and support to be able to listen and relate to users and the public as equals. Investment is needed in an independent infrastructure to provide training, support and accountability for user members on committees. Paying expenses and loss of earnings for user members on committees is also important: they are often the only members of a committee who are expected to give their time voluntarily. This finance is important both to enable people to participate and to indicate that their contribution is valued as much as the other highly paid members of such committees. The concepts of 'lay people' and 'experts' need to be redefined to give value to the experiences and skills of users.

The government needs to recognize and value the importance of an independent public voice. At national level an independently funded forum of voluntary organizations could be established to promote and co-ordinate users' views, covering all aspects of health and social care, in which groups can give their views without fear of losing their funding – as has been developed in Australia and the Netherlands (Chapter 7).

Also at national level, all citizens should have the opportunity to be involved in debates about ethical issues. These include definitions of when life begins and ends; priorities; and issues about access and who benefits from the way that health care is distributed. These are issues for citizens rather than for professionals alone. In the UK, unlike other countries such as Denmark and France, there is no forum for public discussion about ethical issues. A central ethics committee with strong lay and user representation could provide a national forum for developing a research strategy and stimulating public debate about ethical issues.

National groups need to be able to participate in international networks and lobbying. International consumer groups have an important role in lobbying governments in other countries and monitoring the implementation of regulations. They will have an increasingly important role in monitoring global trade, and the marketing and supply of pharmaceuticals and health products. Collaboration by patient organizations enables them to share information about treatments, their benefits and side effects, and to lobby for research that meets their needs. Governments need to recognize the importance of an independent consumer lobby and to fund international networks and UK organizations to participate in the work of bodies such as the World Trade Organization.

Standards and protection

Protecting users is likely to be most effective where there is a culture that puts the duty to users before the duty to the profession or the organization. This requires internal systems of audit that are transparent and involve users as equals. In addition, there still needs to be external regulation to ensure that services meet minimum standards and that users are protected, including those in residential care and in private facilities. The National Institute for Clinical Excellence (NICE) and the Commission for Health Improvement provide an important opportunity to work in an open way and include a strong user involvement from the start, accountable to the wider user movement.

In the long term there is a need for a system that combines standards to ensure quality of services with arrangements for individuals who may experience problems in health care. The National Standard Frameworks will be set through the NICE and should enable people to know what to expect and be more confident to bring problems to the attention of managers and the licensing authorities. There is also a need for co-ordination between complaints procedures in order to give people explanations about what has happened during care, accountability so that the cause of the problem is identified and dealt with, and arrangements for compensation and redress.

It is also essential that there is recourse to law if standards are not met or if rights are infringed. An important change in the law would permit groups to take legal action where their rights had been infringed or they have been damaged, for example by treatment or taking a drug. It would open up access to justice if more organizations were able to take legal action to protect the interests of people they represent.

Rights and responsibilities

The Patient's Charter in 1991 was an important landmark that gave users more power and made them aware of it. But at the same time it antagonized staff by its confrontational approach, which gave patients rights without specifying their responsibilities. There was a backlash and the emphasis shifted towards stressing patients' responsibilities.

What is the future for charters and rights for users? Rights and responsibilities for patients need to be seen in the context of the rights and responsibilities of citizens, maintaining the difficult balance between respect for the individual and the public interest. In some countries consumer groups are campaigning for comprehensive legislation on patients' rights. In Denmark, patients' rights are spread over 55 acts and ministerial orders so that information is inaccessible to users. Patients' organizations are campaigning for these to be joined in one Act: the Patients' Constitution (Reissmann, 1996). In Finland there is a Patients' Rights Law, passed in 1992, after twenty years of campaigning by consumer groups.

Developing rights to fair treatment has been an approach explored by the Institute for Public Policy Research (Bynoe, 1997). Rights to fair treatment are based on principles recognized in common law and standards for good public administration. They recognize that people should:

1 know the criteria by which they are judged eligible for a service;
2 have their views taken into account in deciding about access or planning provision to meet their needs;
3 expect decisions to be fair and unbiased;
4 receive clear reasons for decisions taken about them;
5 have the decision reviewed if they object to it;
6 expect redress if rights are not enforced.

In health care, however, the critical question is not just eligibility for a service, but how people make decisions about what service or treatment is best. In order to take on responsibility for decisions, people need access to independent information, and to be respected and trusted to make their own decisions. If you are thinking of having an operation or procedure with serious long-term consequences, it is sensible to ask for a second opinion and these need to be readily available. Publication of information on mortality rates after treatment and the skills and experience of consultants is promoted by user groups, but until recently it was strongly opposed by the medical profession. However, unless information about outcomes and success rates is widely known, there is no incentive for standards to improve or for managers to take action to protect patients from less skilled practitioners.

Health care and health policy

What might a health service planned by users look like? Based on the policies developed by voluntary groups and research of users' views, the sort of health services that would meet the requirements of users are considered below in relation to people with asthma, mental health problems, eating disorders, maternity services and breast cancer.

Asthma

Asthma is a clinical mystery. It has increased by between twenty and sixty per cent over the past twenty-five years, as part of a general increase in allergies. One in seven children is thought to be suffering from asthma, double the rate of ten years ago. The reasons for this epidemic are not clearly understood. The environment is largely blamed – the indoor environment (tobacco smoke, house dust mites, cooking stove gases and pets) and the outdoor environment (emissions from vehicles, industry and pollens). Now there is a suggestion that antibiotics may be impli-cated. If antibiotics are given to young children they may deplete bacteria in the gut and have an effect on the normal development of the immune system. Though the causes are not accurately pinpointed, they are recog-nized to be in the environment. However, the main response has been to improve the management of asthma by the use of drugs, carrying out research into drug treatments rather than other approaches. Medication can be effective but only suppresses symptoms – and has side effects. There is need for research into non-drug alternatives.

Services for people with asthma and other chronic conditions need to be integrated between primary care and specialist services, using shared guidelines. A study in Scotland found that patients with asthma and their carers who had experienced integrated care, preferred it (GRASSIC, 1994). The 'disease management' approach that focuses on the individual patient's experience of living with a disease is likely to provide more integrated care, though it may encourage more dependence on drugs rather than other strategies. People with asthma and their carers need information and support, but much of the information produced about managing asthma is funded by the drug companies. A survey by the National Asthma Campaign (1994) found that both professionals and people with asthma wanted independent materials.

Without changes in the environment the increase in asthma is likely to continue. A report from the Parliamentary Office of Science and Technology (1994) blamed the rise partly on increases in vehicle fumes and suggested more monitoring and control in cities to stop people driving when air pollution reaches levels that spark off asthma attacks. There are particular problems in hotter summers when the fumes become more noxious on exposure to sunlight. Organizations representing users need to work more closely with environmental groups to campaign for more monitoring and regulation of environmental pollution at local, national and international levels.

Mental health problems

Developing services for people with mental health problems raises many difficulties. Mental health policies aim to help people in emotional distress while also, where deemed necessary, controlling their behaviour and protecting other people from them. There is a difficult balance between protecting the public from possible violence and ensuring that people with mental health problems do not lose their civil rights. It is important that the public understand mental health problems and respect the rights of individual citizens.

Mental health services have been based on the theory that emotional distress is a biomedical condition for which medical treatments such as drugs, psychosurgery and ECT are appropriate. However, there are many conflicting views among professionals. Some, such as the psychiatrist Thomas Szaz (1970), argue that madness does not exist but is manu-factured by society in response to its own problems and its need to create and persecute outsiders. Others see the origins of mental illness to be in past experiences and the solutions to lie in understanding these and finding new ways of thinking and behaving. Jeffrey Masson (1989), who trained as a Freudian psychoanalyst, has taken an extreme line in *Against Therapy*. He argues that all therapy is inherently abusive because of the imbalance in power between patient and therapist. In so far as he was able to offer an alternative, he suggested the answer may lie in self-help and co-counselling.

Behind theories of mental illness, and the policies based on them, are serious conflicts between professionals themselves and between patients, their carers and professionals. Whatever the truth, users of mental health systems want an holistic approach – support and help in the community with dealing with their problems – not just drugs. They say that drugs are over-rated and overprescribed. They say that side effects are not taken seriously and that management of side effects involves simply prescribing more drugs to counteract them – drugs which, in turn, have their own side effects.

People with mental health problems face very different difficulties when they live in the community than when they live in hospital. In hospital, food, housing, social relationships, support and entertainment are provided for an individual, though they may not be of their choosing. Out of hospital, they need somewhere to live, an income, a varied social life, employment, help and support, respect and trust, choice and to be consulted (Mental Health Foundation, 1994). When patients stay in hospital the side effects of drugs, such as loss of concentration, loss of memory, shaking and jerky movements, do not have such serious consequences as they do in the community where they interfere with the ability to cope, while also increasing the stigma and vulnerability patients feel, as well as the prejudice they meet from other people.

Rogers and colleagues (1993) describe two possible future scenarios for providing mental health services. There is a 'nightmare' scenario where the existing model of psychiatric services is transferred to the community as the big psychiatric hospitals close down. This would favour physical treatment in hospital settings, forcing people to have treatment that they may not want and separating mentally ill people from others. This scenario would involve resources being split between the old 'asylums', new acute psychiatric units and local authority community care initiatives. No single agency would have responsibility or be resourced adequately. The 'revolving door' policies of the 1980s would continue as some people were admitted in crisis to hospital and then returned to the community, with inadequate housing and little support, until the next crisis. Registers of mentally ill people would be kept, and surveillance and enforced treatment would be part of the 'management' of people discharged from hospital. The public would be concerned about controlling people with severe mental health problems who may be potentially violent. Mental health services would remain dominated by the medical model.

An alternative scenario is to move away from the 'illness' model of mental health and base mental health services in the community, not in hospitals. If mental health services reflected the views of users, physical and pharmacological treatments would be reduced and more importance would be given to meeting their psychological needs. It would be recognized that recovery from mental health problems depends on the opportunities people have in terms of housing, income and employment as well as their social contacts and support. The emphasis would be upon respecting users' autonomy and citizenship in society. Support, advocacy and self-advocacy projects would be set up by the voluntary sector to provide mutual aid and overnight crisis centres in a way that reflected the needs of people from different ethnic and cultural groups. A user-led mental health service would require changes in public policy to increase the availability of housing, the removal of discrimination in employment and a review of social security benefits.

This would mean a major change in the education and training of mental health workers. Many professionals are pessimistic about the outlook for patients and this pessimism creates problems for users reintegrating into mainstream life. Peter Barham (1997) has argued that the problem of reintegration is not always so much that users do not want to work or that employers are hostile, but the pessimism and low expectations that professionals have of people with mental health problems.

Though the focus would be on 'talking therapies' and advocacy, there would still be an important role for psychiatrists as physicians in monitoring drugs and liaising with clinicians in other specialties. Drugs will still be important for some people, but would be given as part of a wider programme of help.

Mental health would be seen as something that is affected by life circumstances, including income, employment and housing. The importance of helping people cope with their lives in times of difficulty would be recognized, in particular for families with young children, vulnerable young people and refugees. Moving away from the 'illness' model might help people to feel they could ask for help without worrying about being 'labelled' or simply being offered drugs.

Eating disorders

Like other mental health problems, there are many factors that may contribute to someone developing an eating disorder, including personal, family, social, cultural and genetic factors. Eating disorders are not primarily about food. Starving or binge eating are symptoms of an underlying emotional and psychological distress. They are different from other mental illness because most psychiatric drugs are not considered appropriate. Forcing people to eat or stop exercising against their will may hinder rather than help their recovery in the long term, as experience has shown. Consequently there is often no alternative to providing staff-intensive supportive therapies for people with eating disorders. A survey of members of the Eating Disorders Association found that people rated self-help groups as the most helpful, followed by counselling and psychotherapy. Many people considered that the more intrusive approaches, such as medication and behaviour therapy, were unhelpful or made the situation worse (Newton et al., 1993).

People who have had an eating disorder, and their carers, want the fashion and media industries to stop glamorizing skinny women. They also want help available before a serious problem is established. However, people with eating disorders are often very good at disguising their eating and other problems from friends and family. School and primary care workers need to know the signs to look out for and understand how they can best offer help (Hogg, 1995).

Even when the problem is recognized, people with severe eating disorders are often reluctant to accept help, since changing their behaviour is so distressing for them. For most people with eating disorders, outpatient treatment is more effective than in-patient treatment. A study found that in-patients with anorexia nervosa gained weight more rapidly than outpatients, but that this gain did not last; over five years, the best outcome was with outpatient treatment (Crisp et al., 1991). Specialist services are needed for a few people, in particular those who have additional problems, such as drug and alcohol misuse or self-mutilation.

Recovery is a slow process and trust has to be built up in a long-term and continuous relationship with a therapist who understands the feelings of people with eating disorders. People need to be able to change at their own pace in a way that feels safe for them. They require long-term help near where they live, where family and friends can be involved. As they recover, people with eating disorders need the same access to housing, benefits and social support as other people recovering from mental health problems.

Maternity services

User organizations, such as AIMS and the National Childbirth Trust (NCT), have campaigned for the de-medicalization of childbirth, and choice for women in where and how they give birth (Chapter 6). Services that follow from these principles would mean that each woman has a choice in where she gives birth, how she gives birth, in the pain relief used, and who is with her during labour – a midwife or a doctor. Her choice would be respected and staff would work together to support her and ensure that the birth is as safe as possible. In low tech birth centres, women would be admitted to comfortable rooms with en suite bathrooms that ensured privacy and the dedicated attention of the one midwife who has provided most of her antenatal care (Moorhead, 1996). Midwives have had independent practitioner status since the 1902 Midwives Act and would again be respected as practitioners in their own right and specialists in normal birth. After the birth, there would be support and advice to parents to help them cope with caring for a newborn baby and with the adjustments in family life, integrated with other networks of community support.

The changes proposed in the government's *Changing Childbirth* support this vision of maternity services (Chapter 7). In spite of this, the trends are still towards more intervention and medical management in childbirth. This indicates the real and not always overt obstacles to change that exist within health care professions. The key issue for maternity services is safety and avoiding unnecessary medical interventions, while respecting the individual woman's right to autonomy and to make her own decisions. However, the issue of how low tech or midwife births can be made safer has been turned into an issue about consumer choice. Elective Caesarean sections, where there is no medical reason, continue – with some obstetricians and women supporting them as a consumer 'right'. More and more antenatal screening tests are available and more are being developed, though none, including ultrasound which is so popular, have been proved to be of clinical benefit or even safe for the mother or the baby. So, despite government moves to provide local antenatal care in community clinics, women will still have to travel to hospitals where the sophisticated antenatal tests are provided.

Breast cancer

When people find out that they have cancer, their first thought is how to survive, then how to cope with living with a disease which may be contained but is rarely cured, and, finally, how to die. Fear of cancer is so deep-seated that until recently people were not told that they had cancer; even now some doctors prefer euphemisms such as 'non-benign tumour'. There is no cure for most cancers, including breast cancer. Treatment involving different types of surgery, radiotherapy at different doses and chemotherapy can improve survival. If you are treated in a specialist centre, this can make a great difference to survival for breast cancer. The *Calman/Hine Report* proposed that cancer units should be of sufficient size to have multi-disciplinary expert teams to treat the more common cancers and that specialist cancer centres should be based in larger hospitals to treat less common cancers and to support networks of cancer units (Department of Health, 1995).

As far as it goes, the *Calman/Hine Report* reflects users' views by working to ensure access for everyone to the best and state-of-the-art treatment. The report also stressed the importance of psychosocial aspects of cancer and of involving patients in their own care, but did not include any recommendations about this. People with breast cancer want as much information as possible about their cancer, their treatment options, the likelihood of treatment being successful and possible side effects. Understanding complex information and absorbing its implications takes time, especially given the dramatic nature of cancer. They need to build up a rapport with health professionals in order to have a working relationship and participate usefully in discussions about treatment (National Cancer Alliance, 1996). After the initial stage is over, people need practical help. A MORI (1992) survey found that, in terms of day-to-day living, 43 per cent of people with cancer were unable to do all the things that they could do before they were diagnosed and needed help. These included looking after children, cleaning, lifting heavy objects and caring for partners.

Women are very concerned about preventing breast cancer – and, in particular, in protecting their daughters. However, traditional services have concentrated on preventing breast cancer by early diagnosis or even such treatment as Tamoxifen or prophylactic mastectomies. Screening does not prevent cancer: it is early diagnosis and involves risks.

As more evidence emerges about environmental causes of cancer, such as pesticides and pollutants, user groups may see commercial interests as more sinister and wish to campaign against them. These campaigns will need to be undertaken at a national and international level. Heather Goodare (1997) of the UK Breast Cancer Coalition sums this up:

> The kind of issues I hear women give priority to are not more and more Tamoxifen, or comparisons of various chemotherapy regimes. They want to know how to prevent breast cancer in their daughters, what environmental

factors are at work to make the incidence of breast cancer rise so dramatically in developed countries. They ask why in a council estate of 80 houses there have been 25 recent cases of breast cancer: could this be because the estate was built on an old landfill site? . . . They are concerned about factory farming, growth hormones in cattle, the spraying of Lindane from helicopters in East Anglia and South Yorkshire and its apparent link with a rise in breast cancer, environmental oestrogens and so on. (Goodare, 1997)

Conclusions

In looking at health policy and health services from the perspective of users, several themes have run throughout this book. First, there is a real dilemma between our need for hope and the need to learn from the past. Users have rejected some of the myths outlined in Chapter 8, but cling on to some others. They may reject paternalism and want the benefits of consumerism, but continue to expect effective treatment and to believe in the certainty of medicine and medical progress. While people can understand the uncertainty of medicine intellectually, they may be reluctant to accept it emotionally when it affects them and the people they care about. Health care planned by users is not a formula for 'rationality' any more than policy led by the medical profession or the market.

Secondly, where are the boundaries between medicine and health? For example, when is childbirth an abnormal event? When does emotional distress or stress become a mental illness? When should an abnormal cervical smear be treated as if it is cancer? These are areas of constant negotiation and battles among professionals, and between users and professionals. The medicalization of 'health' as well as illness is a threat to people's autonomy, turning them into 'patients' and requiring compliance.

Thirdly, who are the experts? Who should make decisions – whether for the individual or the public good? What legitimacy is there for the powers that now exist to make sure people act in their own best interest? The conflict between paternalism and consumerism persists. It is important to all of us to feel that we are in control of our lives and can make our own decisions. Sometimes the decisions people make may not seem the 'right' ones to professionals, but it is they who live with the consequences of these decisions not professionals. The circumstances where 'compliance' is in the interests of public health are few and need to be clearly defined.

Fourthly, health care is not isolated from other aspects of life. When you or a family member becomes ill, you face many other problems. You may lose your job and your income, your social and family relationships may be affected, your housing may no longer be suitable. Compared to these problems, the immediate symptoms of your illness may seem less important. Campaigning on health issues must be allied to campaigning for better housing, against discrimination, poverty and for a cleaner environment.

Finally, users, carers and the general public may have different interests and they are often divided. These differences mean that users underestimate the common interests they share, which works to the advantage of powerful professional and commercial interests. Users need to recognize how much they do share and build alliances.

The views of users and citizens have had little influence on health policies. Winning the ideological war by, for example, getting views accepted as government policy, still may not achieve the objectives – as campaigners for maternity and children's services know so well. There are powerful interests which have better access to resources and to decision makers, often working in secret to influence public policy. Commercial companies have an interest in focusing health policy on health services, 'cures' and health promoting products – and in attributing the causes of ill health to individual behaviour, rather than to wider environmental, economic or social causes.

A stronger voice for users might not solve the problem of escalating costs or increasing demand. People may want a comprehensive system but be reluctant to pay for it. Users, carers and the general public may prefer the hope and promises offered by treatment and medicines, and make demands that are not based on evidence. Many people may prefer a health system based on hope rather than evidence. But health policies that are open to public accountability, in which citizens and users have a strong voice, are likely to lead to a healthier society where health is put before health care and commercial interests. Patients would become citizens with the rights and responsibilities that this entails.

REFERENCES

ACHCEW (1991) *Community Health Council Core Activities.* London: Association of CHCs for England and Wales.

ACHCEW (1996) *The Patients' Agenda: What the Patient's Charter Leaves Out – the Rights you Don't yet Have in the NHS.* London: Association of CHCs for England and Wales.

ACHCEW and AVMA (1992) *A Health Standards Inspectorate: A Proposal.* London: Association of CHCs for England and Wales.

Action for Sick Children (Scotland) (1995) *Parental Access and Family Facilities in Wards Admitting Children in Scotland: 1995 Update on the Survey Carried Out in 1985.* Edinburgh: Action for Sick Children (Scotland).

Adami, H., Baron, J.A. and Rothman, K.J. (1994) 'Ethics of a prostate cancer screening trial', *The Lancet*, 343: 958–960.

Adams, J. (1995) 'With complements', *Health Service Journal*, 1 June: 23.

Advisory Council on the Misuse of Drugs (1984) *Prevention.* London: HMSO.

Agass, M., Coulter, A., Mant, D. and Fuller, A. (1991) 'Patient participation in general practice: who participates?', *British Journal of General Practice*, 41: 198–201.

Age Concern. (1996) *Not At My Age: Why the Present Breast Screening System is Failing Women Aged 65 and Over.* London: Age Concern.

Age Concern (1997) *Health care for Older People: the Ageism Issue.* London: Age Concern.

Ahmed, T. and Webb-Johnson, A. (1995) 'Voluntary groups', in S. Fernando (ed.), *Mental Health in a Multi-ethnic Society.* London: Routledge.

AIMS and NCT (1997) *A Charter for Ethical Research in Maternity Care.* London: Association for Improvements in the Maternity Services.

AIS (1991) 'News Release'. London: Action and Information on Sugars.

AIS (1993a) International Conference on Nutrition: why and how 'sugars' were omitted. News release. London: Action and Information on Sugars.

AIS (1993b) 'News release'. London: Action and Information on Sugars.

AIS (1994) 'News release'. London: Action and Information on Sugars.

Akehurst, R. (1992) 'Presentation', in R. Wiles (ed.), *A Health Service for London: Conference Report.* London: GLACHC.

Alderson, P. (1990) *Choosing for Children: Parents' Consent to Surgery.* Oxford: Oxford University Press.

Allard, A. (1996) 'Involving young people – empowerment or exploitation?', *Children and Society*, 10 (2): 165–167.

Allsop, J. and Mulcahy, L. (1996) *Regulating Medical Work: Formal and Informal Controls.* Buckingham: Open University Press.

Alzheimer's Disease Society (1997) *Experiences of Care in Residential and Nursing Homes.* London: Alzheimer's Disease Society.

Angell, M. (1997) 'The ethics of clinical research in the Third World', *New England Journal of Medicine*, 337 (12): 847–849.

Armstrong, D. (1995) 'The rise of surveillance medicine', *Sociology of Health and Illness*, 17 (3): 393–404.

Audit Commission (1993) *What Seems to be the Matter: Communication between Hospitals and Patients*. London: HMSO.

Audit Commission (1994) *A Prescription for Improvement: Towards More Rational Prescribing in General Practice*. London: HMSO.

Audit Commission (1995) *Setting the Records Straight: A Study of Hospital Medical Records*. London: HMSO.

Audit Commission (1996) *What the Doctor Ordered*. London: HMSO,

Audit Commission (1997) *First Class Delivery: Improving Maternity Services in England and Wales*. London: HMSO.

Austoker, J. (1994) 'Screening and self examination in breast cancer', *British Medical Journal*, 309: 168–174.

Avery, N., Drake, M. and Laing, T. (1993) *Cracking the Codex: An Analysis of Who Sets World Food Standards*. London: National Food Alliance.

Baby Milk Action (1997a) 'Cow and Gate cardigans', *Update*, 21: 9.

Baby Milk Action (1997b) '. . . And breastfeeding counsellors leave', *Update*, 21: 4.

BACCH (1995) *Child Health Rights: Implementing the UN Convention on the Rights of the Child Within the Health Service*. London: British Association for Community Child Health.

Bailar, J.C. and Gornik, H.L. (1997) 'Cancer undefeated', *New England Journal of Medicine*, 336 (22): 1569–74.

Baine, S., Bennington, J. and Russell, J. (1992) *Changing Europe: Challenges Facing the Voluntary and Community Sectors in the 1990s*. London: NCVO Publications and the Community Development Foundation.

Balogh, R. (1996) 'Exploring the role of localities in health commissioning: a review of the literature', *Social Policy and Administration*, 30 (2): 99–113.

Balogh, R. and Bond, S. (1995) 'Telling it like it is', *Health Service Journal*, 16 March: 26–27.

Barclay, S. (1996) *Jaymee: The Story of Child B*. London: Viking.

Barham, P. (1997) *Closing the Asylum: The Mental Patient in Modern Society*. London: Penguin.

Batt, S. (1994) *Patient No More: The Politics of Breast Cancer*. London: Scarlet Press.

Bawdon, F. (1997) 'No cash, no chance?', *Health Service Journal*, 20 November: 7.

Beaumont, P. (1993) *Pesticides, Policies and People*. London: The Pesticides Trust.

Beech, B.A.L. (1997) 'Court ordered Caesareans – a hidden abuse', *AIMS (Association for Improvements in the Maternity Services) Journal*, 8 (3): 1–4.

Beech, B.A.L. (1998) 'Maintaining the myth of Caesarean safety', *AIMS (Association for Improvements in the Maternity Services) Journal*, 9 (4): 1–3.

Beecher, C. and Coochey, C. (1997) 'Had a nice day?', *Health Service Journal*, 21 August: 28–29.

Bennet, G. (1987) *The Wound and the Doctor: Health, Technology and Power in Modern Medicine*. London: Secker and Warburg.

Benster, R. and Pollock, A.M. (1993) 'Guidelines for local research ethics committees: distinguishing between patient and population research in the multi-centre research project', *Public Health*, 107 (1): 3–7.

Benzeval, M. and Judge, K. (1996) 'Access to health care in England: continuing inequalities in the distribution of Gps', *Journal of Public Health Medicine*, 18 (1): 33–40.

Beresford, P. and Croft, S. (1993) *Citizen Involvement: A Practical Guide for Change.* Basingstoke: Macmillan.

Bero, L.A. and Rennie, D. (1996) 'Influences on the quality of published drug studies', *International Journal of Technology Assessment in Health Care*, 12 (2): 209–237.

Besley, T., Hall, J. and Preston, I. (1996) *Private Health Insurance and the State of the NHS.* London: Institute for Fiscal Studies.

Beveridge Report (1942) *Social Insurance and Allied Services.* London: HMSO.

Black and Ethnic Community Care Forum (1992) *Community Care: the Newham Black Experience.* London: Community Involvement Unit.

Black, D. (1996) 'Glasgow: working together to make a healthier city', *World Health*, 49 (1): 22–23.

Black Report (1980) *Inequalities in Health.* London: DHSS.

Blauw, G.J. and Westendorp, R.G.J. (1995) 'Asthma deaths in New Zealand: whodunnit?' *The Lancet*, 345: 2–3.

Blaxter, M. (1990) *Health and Lifestyles.* London: Tavistock/Routledge.

Blaxter, M. (1995) *Consumers and Research in the NHS: Consumer Issues Within the NHS.* London: Department of Health.

Blendon, R.J., Leitman, R., Morrison, I. and Donelan, K. (1990) 'Satisfaction with health systems in ten nations', *Health Affairs*, Summer, 19 (2): 185–192.

Blenkinsopp, A. and Bradley, C. (1996) 'Patients, society, and increase in self medication', *British Medical Journal*, 312: 629–632.

Bolger, M. (1996) 'Medical negligence litigation – a plaintiff's view on the need for change', *Health Care Risk Report*, July / August: 6–9.

Bradburn, J., Maher, J., Adewuyi-Dalton, R., Grunfeld, E., Lancaster, T. and Mant, D. (1995) 'Developing clinical trial protocols: the use of patient focus groups', *Psycho-Oncology*, 4: 107–112.

Breggin, P. (1993) *Toxic Psychiatry.* London: HarperCollins.

Brewin, T. (1997) '"Blanket" consent to trials would be a good idea', *British Medical Journal*, 315: 253.

Brotchie, J. and Wann, M. (1993) *Training for Lay Participation in Health: Token Voices or Champions of the People?* London: Patients Association.

Bruggen, P. (1997) *Who Cares? True Stories of the NHS Reforms.* Charlbury: Jon Carpenter Publishing.

Buck, N., Devlin, H.B. and Lunn, J.N. (1989) *The Report of a Confidential Enquiry into Perioperative Deaths.* London: The Nuffield Provincial Hospitals Trust and The King's Fund.

Buckland, S., Lupton, C. and Moon, G. (1995) *An Evaluation of the Role and Impact of Community Health Councils.* Portsmouth: University of Portsmouth.

Buckley, M. (1997) 'Industrious resolution', *Health Service Journal*, 19 June: 32–33.

Butler, J. (1992) *Patients, Policies and Politics.* Buckingham: Open University Press.

Buttery, Y., Walshe, K., Coles, J. and Bennett, J. (1994) *Evaluating Medical Audit: The Development of Audit.* London: CASPE Research.

Bynoe, I. (1997) *Rights to Fair Treatment.* London: Institute for Public Policy Research.

Byrne P. (1997) *Social Movements in Britain.* London: Routledge.

Cabinet Office (1997) *Your Right to Know: Freedom of Information.* London: Stationery Office.

Campbell, H., Boyd, K.M. and Surry, S.A.M. (1997) 'Journals should require routine reporting of consent rates', *British Medical Journal*, 315: 247.

Carr Hill, R.A. (1991) 'Allocating resources to health care: is the QALY a technical solution to a political problem?', *International Journal of Health Services*, 21 (2): 351–363.

Carr Hill, R.A. (1992) 'The measurement of patient satisfaction', *Journal of Public Health Medicine*, 14: 236–249.

Clarke, A. (1995) 'Population screening for genetic susceptibility to disease', *British Medical Journal*, 311: 35–38.

Coast, J. and Donovan, J. (1996) 'Public participation: an historical perspective' in J. Coast, J. Donovan and S. Frankel (eds), *Priority Setting: The Health Care Debate*. Chichester: Wiley.

College of Health (1994) *Consumer Audit Guidelines*. London: College of Health.

COMA (1989) *The Diets of British School Children*. Committee on Medical Aspects of Food, DHSS Report 36. London: HMSO.

Consumers' Association (1987) 'Making your doctor better', *Which?*, 30: 230–232.

Consumers' Association (1996) 'The drug information gap', *Health Which?*, October, 167–170.

Consumers' Association (1997a) 'On the record', *Health Which?*, August: 136–137.

Consumers' Association (1997b) 'Cause for complaint', *Which?*, September: 15–19.

Consumers' Association (1997c) 'How safe is complementary medicine?' *Health Which?*, October: 160–161.

Consumers' Association, Drugs and Therapeutics Bulletin, National Prescribing Centre (1997) Medicines and the NHS, Part 6. *The Pharmaceutical Industry*. London: Consumers' Association, Drugs and Therapeutics Bulletin, National Prescribing Centre.

Consumers International (1996) *Campaigning for Patients' Rights: A Consumer Action Kit*. London: Consumers International.

Consumers International (1997a) *Genetic Engineering and Food Safety: The Consumer Interests*. London: Consumers International.

Consumers International (1997b) *Position of Consumers International prepared for the Twenty-Second Session of the Codex Alimentarius Commission re: Involvement of Non-governmental Organisations in the Work of the Codex Alimentarius Commission*. London: Consumers International.

Cooper, L., Coote, A., Davies, A. and Jackson, C. (1995) *Voices Off*. London: Institute for Public Policy Research.

Coulter, A. (1994) 'Assembling the evidence: outcomes research', in M. Dunning and G. Needham (eds), *But Will it Work Doctor?: A Report of a Conference about Involving Users in Health Services Outcomes Research*. Consumer Health Information Consortium.

Council of Europe (1994) *Participation by Citizens-consumers in the Management of Local Public Services. Local and Regional Authorities in Europe No. 54*. Strasbourg: Council of Europe.

Coward, R. (1989) *The Whole Truth: The Myth of Alternative Health*. London: Faber and Faber.

Crawford, R. (1985) 'A cultural account of "health": control, release and the social body'; in J.B. McKinlay (ed.), *Issues in the Political Economy of Health Care*. London: Tavistock.

Crisp, A.H., Norton, K., Gowers, S., Halek, C., Bowyer, C., Yelham, D., Levett, G. and Bhat, A. (1991) 'Controlled study of the effect of therapies aimed at adolescent and family psychopathology in anorexia nervosa', *British Journal of Psychiatry*, 159: 325–333.

Dalziel, M. and Garrett, C. (1987) 'Intra-regional variation in treatment of end stage renal failure', *British Medical Journal*, 294: 1382–3.

Davidson, L. (1998) 'Alarm unheard or unheeded?' *Health Service Journal*, 4 June: 14–15.

Dekkers, A.F. (1995) 'Patients' rights in the Netherlands', in WHO, *Promotion of the Rights of Patients in Europe*. The Hague: Kluwer Law International.

Department of Health (1989) *Working for Patients*. London: HMSO.

Department of Health (1991a) *The Patient's Charter*. London: Department of Health.

Department of Health (1991b) *Local Research Ethics Committees*. Health Service Guidance (HSG(91) 5) August.

Department of Health (1992). *The Health of the Nation: A Strategy for Health in England*. London: HMSO.

Department of Health (1993) *Changing Childbirth: Report of the Expert Maternity Group*. London: HMSO.

Department of Health (1994) *Being Heard: the Report of a Review Committee on NHS Complaints Procedures*. London: HMSO.

Department of Health (1995) *A Policy Framework for Commissioning Cancer Services: A Report of the Expert Advisory Group on Cancer to the Chief Medical Officers of England and Wales*. London: Department of Health. (Calman/Hine Report.)

Department of Health (1997a) *The Patient's Charter: Mental Health Services*. London: Department of Health.

Department of Health (1997b) *The New NHS: Modern – Dependable*. London: Stationery Office.

Department of Health (1998a) *A First Class Service: Quality in the New NHS*. London: Department of Health.

Department of Health (1998b) *Our Healthier Nation*. London: Stationery Office.

Department of Health (1998c) *Healthy Living Centres: Report of a Conference held on 2 April 1998*. London: Stationery Office.

DHSS (1976) *Prevention and Health: Everybody's Business*. London: HMSO.

DHSS (1983) *NHS Management Inquiry*. London: DHSS (*Griffiths Report*).

Donovan, J. and Blake, D. (1992) 'Patient compliance: deviance or reasoned decision making?', *Social Science and Medicine*, 34 (5): 507–513.

Dowell, A.C., Ochera, J.J., Hilton, S.R., Bland, J.M., Harris, T., Jones, D.R. and Katbamna, S. (1996) 'Prevention in practice: results of a 2 year follow up of routine health promotion interventions in general practice', *Family Practice*, 13 (4): 357–362.

Dowie, R. (1995) 'Health services research in the United Kingdom 1990–92', *Journal of Public Health Medicine*, 17 (1): 93–97.

Dowson, S. (1990) *Keeping It Safe: Self Advocacy by People with Learning Difficulties and the Professional Response*. London: Values into Action.

Doyal, L., Epstein, S.S., Gee, D., Green, K., Irwin, A., Russell, D., Steward, F. and Williams, R. (1983) *Cancer in Britain: The Politics of Prevention*. London: Pluto Press.

Doyle, M. (1997) 'The legal importance of living wills', *British Journal of Health Care Management*, 3 (5): 270–272.

Dunnell, K. (1995) 'Population review: (2) are we healthier?', *Population Trends*, 82: 12–18.

Earl-Slater, A. (1997). 'Regulating the price of the UK drugs: second thoughts after the government's first report', *British Medical Journal*, 314: 365–368.

EC (1996) *The State of Health in the European Community: First Public Health Report*. Brussels: European Commission.

Edwards, N. (1996) 'Lore unto themselves', *Health Service Journal*, 12 September: 26–27.

EMEA (1997) *Interim Report on the Consultation Exercise on Transparency and Access to documents at the EMEA*. London: The European Agency for the Evaluation of Medicinal Products.

Enkin, M., Keirse, M.J.N.C. and Chalmers, I. (1992) *A Guide to Effective Care in Pregnancy and Childbirth*. Oxford: Oxford University Press.

EPHA (1995) *Commercial Sponsorship and NGOs*. Brussels: European Public Health Alliance.

Esmail, A. and Everington, S. (1997) 'Asian doctors are still being discriminated against', *British Medical Journal*, 314: 1619.

Fallowfield, F.J., Hall, A., Maguire, G.P. and Baum, M. (1990) 'Psychological outcomes of different treatment policies in women with early cancer outside a clinical trial', *British Medical Journal*, 301: 575–580.

Fallowfield, L. (1997) 'Making decisions about treatments: how do patients with cancer choose?'; in M. Dunning, G. Needham, and S. Weston, (eds), *But Will It Work Doctor? Report of a Conference, Northampton 22 and 23 May 1996*. Oxford: But Will It Work, Doctor? Group.

Farrant, W. and Russell, J. (1986) *The Politics of Health Information: Beating Heart Disease as a Case Study in HEC Publications*. London: Bedford Way Papers, 28, Institute of Education, London University.

Faulder, C. (1985) *Whose Body Is It? The Troubling Issue of Informed Consent*. London: Virago.

Fentiman, I.S., Tirelli, U., Monfardini, S., Schneider, M., Festen, J., Cognetti, F. and Aapro, M.S. (1990) 'Cancer in the elderly: why so badly treated?', *The Lancet*, 335 (8696): 1020–1022.

Fernando, S. (1995) 'Social realities and mental health', in S. Fernando, (ed.), *Mental Health in a Multi-ethnic Society*. London: Routledge.

Fisher, P. and Ward, A. (1994) 'Complementary medicine in Europe', *British Medical Journal*, 309: 107–109.

Fitzpatrick, R. and Bolton, M. (1994) 'Qualitative methods for assessing health care', *Quality in Health Care*, 3: 107–113.

Foster, C. (1995) 'Why do research ethics committees disagree with each other?', *Journal of the Royal College of Physicians of London*, 29 (4): 315–318.

Foster, P. (1995) *Women and the Health Care Industry*. Buckingham: Open University Press.

Frankel, M. (1994) 'Restrictions on disclosure', in *Proceedings of a Seminar on Commercial Confidentiality, 18 October*. London: Campaign for Freedom of Information.

Frankel, M. (1996) 'Open and shut case', The *Guardian*, 18 June.

Frater, A. (1992) 'Health outcomes: a challenge to the status quo', *Quality in Health Care*, 1: 87–88.

Freake, D., Crowley, P., Steiner, M. and Drinkwater, C. (1997) 'Local heroes', *Health Service Journal*, 10 July: 28–29.

Garrett, L. (1994) *The Coming Plague: Newly Emerging Diseases in a World Out of Balance*. London: Penguin.

Gaskin, K. and Vincent, J. (1996) *Co-operating for Health: The Potential Contribution of the Co-operative Movement and Community Well-Being Centres to Health of the Nation Activities.* Centre for Research in Social Policy. Loughborough: Loughborough University.

Genn, H. and Genn, Y. (1989) *The Effectiveness of Representation at Tribunals.* London: Lord Chancellor's Department.

Gilbert, D. and Chetley, A. (1996) 'New trends in drug promotion', *Consumer Policy Review*, 6 (5): 162–167.

Gilhooly, L.M. and McGhee, S.M. (1991) 'Medical records: practicalities and principles for patient possession', *Journal of Medical Ethics*, 17: 138–143.

GLACHC (1994) *London's CHCs: A Wealth of Ideas and Activities.* London: Greater London Association of Community Health Councils.

Glenister, D. (1994) 'Patient participation in psychiatric services: a literature review and proposal for a research strategy. *Journal of Advanced Nursing*, 19: 802–811.

GMC (1983) *Professional Conduct and Discipline: Fitness to Practice.* London: General Medical Council.

GMC (1995) *Duties of a Doctor.* London: General Medical Council.

Goodare, H. (1996) *Fighting Spirit: The Stories of Women in the Bristol Breast Cancer Survey.* London: Scarlet Press.

Goodare, H. (1997) 'Is consent truly informed?' in C. Hogg (ed.), *A Voice for the Guinea Pig?* London: Consumers for Ethics in Research.

Goodare, H. and Smith, R. (1995) 'The rights of patients in research', *British Medical Journal*, 310: 1277–8.

Graboys, T., Biegelsen, B., Lampert, S., Blatt, C.M. and Lown, B. (1992) 'Results of a second opinion trial among patients recommended for coronary angiography', *Journal of the American Medical Association*, 268: 2537–40.

GRASSIC (1994) 'Integrated care for asthma: a clinical, social and economic evaluation', *British Medical Journal*, 308: 559–563.

Gravhold, C.H., Svend, J., Naeraa, R.W. and Hansen, J. (1996) 'Prenatal and postnatal prevalence of Turner's Syndrome: a registry study', *British Medical Journal*, 312: 16–21.

Green, D. (1985) *Which Doctor? A Critical Analysis of the Professional Barriers to Competition in Health Care.* London: Institute of Economic Affairs.

Green, D. (1989) *Should Doctors Advertise?* London: Institute of Economic Affairs.

HAI (1997) *Power, Patents and Pills: Seminar Report.* Amsterdam: Health Action International.

Halek, C. (1994) 'Recovery', *Signpost.* December. Norwich: Eating Disorders Association.

Hamilton, K. (1997) *The Health Promoting School: A Summary of the ENHPS Evaluation Project in England.* London: Health Education Authority.

Handy, C. (1988) *Understanding Voluntary Organisations.* London: National Council for Voluntary Organisations.

Harries, U.J., Fentem, P.H., Tuxworth, W. and Hoinville, W. (1994) 'Local research ethics committees: widely differing responses to a national survey protocol', *Journal of the Royal College of Physicians*, 26: 150–154.

Harris, J. (1997). 'The injustice of compensation for victims of medical accidents', *British Medical Journal*, 314: 1821.

Harrison, S., Hunter, D., Johnston, I., Nicholson, N., Thunhurst, C. and Wistow, G. (1991) *Health Before Health Care.* London: Institute for Public Policy Research.

Harvey, B. (1991) 'Pressure groups and policy making in the European Communities'. Paper presented to the Nuffield College Oxford, European Studies Centre, 17–19 May 1991. Quoted in S. Baine, J. Bennington and J. Russell (1992), *Changing Europe: Challenges Facing the Voluntary and Community Sectors in the 1990s*. London: NCVO Publications and the Community Development Foundation.

Hayes, L. and Mintzes, B. (1997) 'The ties that bind: drug industry sponsorship'. *HAI-Lights*, 3 (2–3): 1–3.

Heide, B. van der. (1996) 'Principles, obstacles and solutions for rational drug use', in *Health Care in a Changing World: Patients' Rights and Responsibilities*. London: Consumers International and Slovene Consumers Association.

Hirst, J. (1997) 'A voice for the guinea pig: Consumer involvement a dream or a reality?', in C. Hogg (ed.), *A Voice for the Guinea Pig?*. London: Consumers for Ethics in Research.

Hodgkin, R. (1993) 'Policy review: children and medical treatment', *Children and Society*, 7 (2): 211–213.

Hoffenberg, R. (1987) *Clinical Freedom*. London: Nuffield Provincial Hospital Trust.

Hoffmann, D.E. (1993) 'Evaluating ethics committees: a view from the outside', *The Millbank Quarterly*, 71 (4): 677–701.

Hogbin, B. and Fallowfield, L. (1989) 'Getting it taped: the "bad news" consultation with cancer patients', *British Journal of Hospital Medicine*, 41: 330–333.

Hogg, C. (1989) 'A look backwards and forwards', in C. Hogg and F. Winkler (eds), *Community/Consumer Representation in the NHS*. London: Greater London Association of CHCs.

Hogg, C. (1992) *Centring Excellence: National and Regional Health Services in London*. London: King's Fund Commission on the Future of Acute Services in London.

Hogg, C. (1994) *Beyond the Patient's Charter: Working with Users*. London: Health Rights.

Hogg, C. (1995) *Eating Disorders: A Guide to Commissioning and Providing Services*. Norwich: Eating Disorders Association.

Hogg, C. (1996) *Back From the Margins: Which Future for CHCs?* London: Institute of Health Services Management, Association of Community Health Councils for England and Wales.

Hogg, C., Chadwick, T. and Dale-Perera, A. (1997) *Drug Using Parents*. London: Local Government Drugs Forum.

Holland, W. and Stewart, S. (1990) *Screening in Health Care: Benefit or Bane?* London: Nuffield Provincial Hospitals Trust.

Honigsbaum, F., Holmstrom, S. and Calltrop, J. (1997) *Making Choices for Health Care*. Oxford: Radcliffe Medical Press.

House of Commons Public Service Committee (1996) First Report, Session 1995/96, *The Code of Practice for Public Appointments*. London: HMSO.

House of Commons Select Committee (1996) *Long Term Care: Future Provision and Funding*. London: HMSO.

Howard, W. (1996) *Men's Attitude to Health Checks and Awareness of Male-specific Cancers*. London: Health Education Authority.

Hughes, D. (1991) 'A question of judgement', *Health Services Journal*, 13 June: 22–24.

Hunter, D. (1997) 'A long life for a quick fix?', *Health Service Journal*, 4 September: 22.

Hunter, D.J. (1995) 'Accountability and local democracy', *British Journal of Health Care Management*, 1 (2): 78–81.

IDDT (1997a) Insulin Dependent Diabetes Trust, Summer Newsletter.

IDDT (1997b) *What Patients Need from the Pharmaceutical Industry and Government*. Northampton: Insulin Dependent Diabetes Trust.

IGBM (1997) *Cracking the Code: Monitoring the International Code of Marketing of Breast-milk Substitutes*. London: Interagency Group on Breastfeeding Monitoring.

Illich, I. (1975) *Limits to Medicine – Medical Nemesis: The Expropriation of Health*. London: Marion Boyars.

Insight (1996) *Resourcing and Performance Management in Community Health Councils: Final Report to NHS Executive*. Leeds: Insight Management Consulting.

IOCU (1994a) *A Searching Look at Advertisements*. London: International Organisation of Consumer Unions.

IOCU (1994b) *The Case for Openness: Consultation and Transparency in the World Trade Organisation*. London: International Organisation of Consumer Unions.

Irvine, D. (1997) 'The performance of doctors 1: professionalism and self regulation in a changing world', *British Medical Journal*, 314: 1540–1542.

Jenkins, R. (1991) *Food for Wealth or Health?* London: Socialist Health Association.

Jewkes, R. and Murcott, A. (1998) 'Community representatives: representing the "community"?' *Social Science and Medicine*, 46 (7): 843–858.

Jones, S. (1994) *The Language of Genes*. London: Flamingo.

Joosens, L. and Raw, M. (1996) 'Are tobacco subsidies a misuse of public funds?' *British Medical Journal*, 312: 832–835.

Joule, N. (1992) *User Involvement in Medical Audit: A Spoke in the Wheel or a Link in the Chain*. London: Greater London Association of Community Health Councils.

Joule, N. (1997) *Choices and Opportunities for User Involvement in the Primary Care-led NHS: Exploring Relationships between CHCs and GPs in London*. London: Greater London Association of Community Health Councils.

Kanavos, P. (1996) 'Pharmaceutical consolidation and public policy', *Eurohealth*, 2 (4): 30–32.

Kane, P. (1991) *Women's Health: from Womb to Tomb*. Basingstoke: Macmillan.

Kaplan, S.H., Greenfield, S. and Ware, J.E. (1989) 'Assessing the effects of physician–patient interactions on the outcome of chronic disease', *Medical Care*, 27 (3 supplement): 110–127.

Karpf, A. (1988) *Doctoring the Media*. London: Routledge.

Kelson, M. (1995) *Consumer Involvement Initiatives in Clinical Audit and Outcomes*. London: College of Health.

Kerrigan, D.D., Thevasagayam, R.S., Woods, T.O., McWelch, I., Thomas, W.E.G., Shorthouse, A.J., and Dennison, A.R. (1993) 'Who's afraid of informed consent?', *British Medical Journal*, 306: 298–300.

Kitzhaber, J.A. (1993) 'Rationing in action: prioritising health services in an era of limits: the Oregon experience', *British Medical Journal*, 307: 373–377.

Koopmans, P.P. (1995) 'Registration of drugs for treating cancer and HIV infection: a plea to carry out phase 3 trials before admission to the market', *British Medical Journal*, 310: 1305–6.

Laing's Review of Private Health Care (1997) London: Laing and Buisson Publications Ltd.

Lamb, B., and Percival, R. (1992) *Paying for Disability: No Fault Compensation: Panacea or Pandora's Box?* London: The Spastics Society.

Le Grand, J. (1997) 'Knights, knaves or pawns? Human behaviour and social policy', *Journal of Social Policy*, 26 (2): 149–169.

Leidl, R. and Rhodes, G. (1997) 'Cross-border health care in the European Union', *European Journal of Public Health*, 7 (3) Supplement: 1–3.

Lindow, V. (1991) 'Experts, lies and stereotypes', *Health Service Journal*, 29 August: 18–19.

Lindow, V. and Morris, L. (1995) *Service User Involvement: Synthesis of Findings and Experience in the Field of Community Care*. York: Joseph Rowntree.

Lobstein, T. (1996) 'The cost of food', in C. Hewett, C. Hogg, M. Leicester, and H. Rosenthal, (eds), *Health and the Environment*. London: Socialist Health Association and the Socialist Environment and Resources Association.

Lock, S. and Wells, F. (eds) (1996) *Fraud and Misconduct in Medical Research*. Second edition. London: BMJ Publishing.

Lohmann, L. (1998) 'Whose Voice is Speaking? How Opinion Polling and Cost-Benefit Analysis Synthesizes New "Publics"', *Briefing No. 7*. Sturminster Newton, Dorset: The Corner House.

Long, A.F. (1997) 'The Leeds Declaration: three years on, a symbol or a catalyst for change?', *Critical Public Health*, 7 (1 and 2): 73–81.

Lord Chancellor's Department (1997) *Who Decides? Making Decisions on Behalf of Mentally Incapacitated Adults*. London: Stationery Office.

Lowry, S. and Smith, J. (1992) 'Duplicate publication', *British Medical Journal*, 304: 999–1000.

MAFF (1997) *The Food Standards Agency: A Force for Change*. London: Stationery Office.

Masson, J. (1989) *Against Therapy*. London: Collins.

Maxwell, R. (1997) *An Unplayable Hand? BSE, CJD and the British Government*. London: King's Fund.

McFarlane, A. and Mugford, M. (1992) *Birth Counts: Statistics of Pregnancy and Childbirth*. London: HMSO.

McIver, S. (1993a) *Investing in Patient's Representatives*. Birmingham: National Association of Health Authorities and Trusts.

McIver, S. (1993b) *Obtaining the Views of Users of Primary and Community Health Services*. London: King's Fund Centre.

McPherson, K. (1990) 'International differences in medical care practices', in *Health Care Systems in Transition: The Search for Efficiency*. Paris: OECD.

Meade, T.W. (1994) 'The trouble with ethics committees', *Journal of the Royal College of Physicians*, 28:102–103.

Medewar, C. (1992) *Power and Dependence*. London: Social Audit.

Medewar, C. (1997) 'The antidepressant web: marketing depression and making medicines work', *International Journal of Risk and Safety in Medicine*, 10: 75–126.

Mental Health Act Commission (1995) *Sixth Biennial Report 1993–95*. London: HMSO.

Mental Health Foundation (1994) *Creating Community Care*. London: Mental Health Foundation.

Mental Health Foundation (1997) *Knowing Our Own Minds: A Survey of How People in Emotional Distress Take Control of Their Lives*. London: Mental Health Foundation.

Meredith, P. (1993) 'Patient participation in decision-making and consent to treatment: the case of general surgery', *Sociology of Health and Illness*, 15 (3): 315–336.

Meredith, P., Emberton, M. and Wood, C. (1995) 'New directions in information for patients'. *British Medical Journal*, 311: 4–5.

Middleton, J.F. (1995) 'Asking patients to write lists: a feasibility study', *British Medical Journal*, 311: 34.

Millar, B. (1998) 'In the public interest?', *Health Service Journal*, 14 May: 9.

Milo, N. (1988) 'Public policy as the cornerstone for a new public health: local and global beginnings', *Family and Community Health*, 2: 57–71.

Montgomery, J. (1997) *Health Care Law*. Oxford: Oxford University Press

Moorhead, J. (1996) *New Generations: 40 Years of Birth in Britain*. Cambridge: HMSO and National Childbirth Trust Publishing Ltd.

MORI (1992) *The Social Impact of Cancer*. London: Cancer Relief MacMillan Fund.

MORI (1994) *Evaluation of Bilingual Health Care Schemes in East London: Evaluation Study Conducted for the East London Consortium*. London: East London Consortium.

Mudur, G. (1997) 'Indian research doesn't reflect country's needs', *British Medical Journal*, 315: 271.

Mullen, P. (1995). *Is Health Care Rationing Really Necessary? Discussion Paper 36*. Birmingham: Health Services Management Centre, the University of Birmingham.

Nagel, J., McMahon, K., Barbour, M. and Allen, D. (1992) 'Evaluation of the use and usefulness of telephone consultation in one GP practice', *British Medical Journal*, 305: 1266–68.

National Association of Health Authorities and Trusts (1993) *Complaints Do Matter: A Consultative Paper on Future NHS Complaints Arrangements*. Birmingham: National Association of Health Authorities and Trusts.

National Asthma Campaign / Access Options Ltd (1994) *Asthma Perceptions and Treatment: A Survey of Medical Practitioners*. London: National Asthma Campaign.

National Audit Office (1992) *Cervical and Breast Screening in England*. London: HMSO.

National Cancer Alliance (1996) *Patient-centred Cancer Services? What Patients Say*. Oxford: National Cancer Alliance.

Nazroo, J.Y. (1997) *The Health of Britain's Ethnic Minorities*. London: Policy Studies Institute.

NCC (1991) *Pharmaceuticals: A Consumer Perspective*. London: National Consumer Council.

NCC (1993) *It's OK to Complain*: London: National Consumer Council.

NCC (1994a) *Consumer Representation in the Public Sector: How MAFF and the Benefits Agency Consult Users*. London: National Consumer Council.

NCC (1994b) *Secrecy and Medicines in Europe*. London: National Consumer Council.

NCC (1995) *Human Genetics Research: Exploring Some Consumer Concerns*. London: National Consumer Council.

NCC (1997) *NHS Complaints Procedures: The First Year*. London: National Consumer Council.

Nesse, R.M., and Williams, G.C. (1995) *Evolution and Healing: The New Science of Darwinian Medicine*. London: Weidenfeld and Nicolson.

Neuberger, J. (1992) *Ethics and Health Care: The Role of Research Ethics Committees in the United Kingdom*. London: King's Fund Institute.

New, B. (1996) *The Rationing Agenda in the NHS*. London: King's Fund Publishing.

Newton, T., Robinson, P. and Hartley, P. (1993) 'Treatment for Eating Disorders in the United Kingdom. Part II – Experiences of Treatment: A Survey of Members of the Eating Disorders Association', *Eating Disorders Review*, 1 (2): 4–9.

NHSE (1994) *Guidelines for a Local Charter for Users of Mental Health Services*. London: Mental Health Task Force User Group, Department of Health.

NHSE (1995) *Code of Practice on Openness in the NHS*. Leeds: NHS Executive.

NHSE (1996a) *Clinical Audit in the NHS: Using Clinical Audit in the NHS*. London: Department of Health.

NHSE (1996b) *Patient Partnership: Building a Collaborative Strategy*. London: Department of Health.

NHSE (1996c) *Maternity Services Liaison Committees: Guidelines for Working Effectively*. London: Department of Health.

NHSE, Institute of Health Services Management, NHS Confederation (1998) *In the Public Interest: Developing a Strategy for Public Participation in the NHS*. London: Department of Health.

NHSME (1990). *Access to Health Records 1990: A Guide for the NHS*. London: NHS Management Executive.

NHSME (1992) *Local Voices: The Views of Local People in Purchasing for Health*. London: Department of Health.

Nicholson, R. (1997) 'Editorial', *Bulletin of Medical Ethics*, 132: 1–2.

Nolan, Lord (1995) *Standards in Public Life*. London: HMSO.

Novak, R. (1995) 'New push to reduce maternal mortality in poor countries'. *Science*, 269: 780–782.

O'Keefe, E. (1991) 'WHO strategies for Europe: racism and the Alma Ata declaration', *Critical Public Health*, 1: 36–41.

O'Keefe, E. (1993) *Divided London: Towards a European Public Health Approach*. London: University of North London Press.

O'Keefe, E. (1995a) 'Values and ethical issues', in S. Pike and D. Forster (eds), *Health Promotion for All*. Edinburgh: Churchill Livingstone.

O'Keefe, E. (1995b) 'The World Bank: health policy, poverty and equity', *Critical Public Health*, 6 (3): 28–35.

O'Keefe, E. (1996) 'Human rights and health promotion in Europe: the case of children in the United Kingdom', in M. Parker (ed.), *Ethics and Community*. Preston: University of Central Lancashire Press.

Oakley, A. (1989) 'Smoking in pregnancy: smokescreen or risk factor? towards a materialist analysis', *Sociology of Health and Illness*, 11 (4): 311–335.

OECD (1992) 'The Reform of Health Care: A Comparative Analysis of Seven OECD Countries', *Health Policy Studies No. 2*. Paris: OECD.

OECD (1995) 'New Directions in Health Care Policy', *Health Policy Studies No. 7*. Paris: OECD.

Office for National Statistics (1997) *Birth Statistics 1995*. London: Stationery Office.

Office of Fair Trading (1996) *Health Insurance*. London: Office of Fair Trading.

OHE (1997) *Hospital Acquired Infection*. London: Office of Health Economics.

Oliver, S. (1997) 'Involving consumers in generating new evidence', in M. Dunning, G. Needham and S. Weston (eds), *But Will It Work Doctor? Report of a Conference, Northampton 22 and 23 May 1996*. Oxford: But Will It Work, Doctor? Group.

Oliver, S. and Buchanan, P. (1997) *Examples of Lay Involvement in Research and Development*. London: Social Science Research Unit, London University Institute of Education.

Oliver, S.R. (1995) 'How can health service users contribute to the NHS R&D programme?' *British Medical Journal*, 310: 1318–20.

Parliamentary Commissioner for Administration, (1996) *Annual Report for 1995*. London: HMSO.

Parliamentary Office of Science and Technology (1994) *Breathing in Our Cities*. London: HMSO.

Parliamentary Select Committee (1988) *Priorities in Medical Research*. London: HMSO.

Parsons, T. (1970) *The Social System*. London: Routledge Kegan Paul.

Payer, L. (1990) *Medicine and Culture: Notions of Health and Sickness*. London: Gollancz.

Pearn, J. (1995) 'An ethical imperative', *British Medical Journal*, 310: 1313–15.

Petersen, A. and Lupton, D. (1996) *The New Public Health: Health and Self in the Age of Risk*. London: Sage.

Petticrew, M., McKee, M. and Jones, J. (1993) 'Coronary artery surgery: are women discriminated against?' *British Medical Journal*, 306: 1164–6.

Pfeffer, N. (1995) 'What the NHS needs are quasi-people, says CHC chair', *The IHSM Network*, 2 (21): 1.

Pfeffer, N. and Coote, A. (1991) *Is Quality Good for You?* London: Institute for Public Policy Research.

Pharmaceutical Industry Council (1997) *Pharmaceutical Industry Manifesto: What Industry Needs from Government*. London: Pharmaceutical Industry Council.

Pietroni, P. (1996) 'The integrated community care practice: general practice, citizenship and community care', in G. Meads (ed.), *Future Options for General Practice*. Oxford: Radcliffe Medical.

Plant, R. (1989) *Can There Be a Right to Healthcare?* Southampton: Institute of Health Policy Studies, Faculty of Social Sciences, University of Southampton.

Platt Report (1959) *The Welfare of Children in Hospital*. London: HMSO.

Popova, L. (1996) *'Problems of inappropriate drug exports and donations'*, in *Health Care in a Changing World: Patients' Rights and Responsibilities*. London: Consumers International and Slovene Consumers Association.

Porter, R. (1997) *Greatest Benefit to Mankind: A Medical History of Humanity from Antiquity to the Present*. London: HarperCollins.

Posner, T. and Vessey, M. (1988) *Prevention of Cervical Cancer: The Patient's View*. London: King Edward's Hospital Fund for London.

Power, M. (1994) *The Audit Explosion*. London: Demos.

Pritchard, P. (1993) *Involving Patients in General Practice: A Practical Guide to Starting a Patient Participation Group*. London: Royal College of General Practitioners.

Pycock, C.J., King, A. and Marshall, A.J. (1995) 'Management of heart disease in the elderly in the Plymouth health district', *Journal of the Royal College of Physicians of London*, 29 (1): 15–19.

Raffle, A.E., Alden, B. and Mackenzie, E.F.D. (1995) 'Detection rates for abnormal cervical smears: what are we screening for?' *The Lancet* 345: 1469–73.

RAGE National (1997) 'All treatment and trials must have informed consent', *British Medical Journal*, 314: 1134–35.

Refugee Council (1997) *The Health Concerns of Asylum Seekers and Refugees*. London: Refugee Council.

Reissmann, M. (1996) *'Why legislate for patients' rights'*, in *Health Care in a Changing World: Patients' Rights and Responsibilities*. London: Consumers International and Slovene Consumers Association.

Richter, J. (1998) Engineering of Consent: Uncovering Corporate PR. Briefing No. 6. Sturminster Newton, Dorset: The Corner House.

Ridley, M. (1994) *The Red Queen: Sex and the Evolution of Human Nature*. London: Penguin Books.

Riis, P. (1993) 'Medical ethics and the European Community', *Journal of Medical Ethics* 19: 7–12.

Robbins, D. (1990) 'Voluntary organisations and the social state in the European Community', *Voluntas*, 1 (2): 98–128.

Robinson, J. (1988) *A Patient Voice at the GMC: A Lay Member's View at the GMC*. London: Health Rights.

Robinson, J. (1995) 'Why mothers fought obstetricians', *British Journal of Midwifery*, 3 (10): 557–558.

Rock, A.J. (1995) 'Court-ordered obstetrical intervention: a short history', *AIMS (Association for Improvements in the Maternity Services) Journal*, 7 (3): 6–8.

Rogers, A., Pilgrim, D. and Lacey, R. (1993) *Experiencing Psychiatry: Users Views of Services*. London: MIND.

Rosenthal, M. (1992) 'Medical discipline in cross cultural perspective: the United States, Britain and Sweden', in R. Dingwall and P. Fenn (eds), *Quality and Regulation in Health Care: International Experiences*. London: Routledge.

Rosenthal, M. (1995) *The Incompetent Doctor: Behind Closed Doors*. Buckingham: Open University Press.

Rosleff, F. and Lister, G. (1995) *European Healthcare Trends: Towards Managed Care in Europe*. London: Coopers and Lybrand.

Rovelli, M., Palmeri, D., Vossler, E., Bartus, S., Hull, D. and Schweizer, R. (1989) 'Non-compliance in organ transplant recipients', *Transplantation Proceedings*, 21 (1): 833–834. Quoted in Royal Pharmaceutical Society of Great Britain (1997) *From Compliance to Concordance: Achieving Shared Goals in Medicine Taking*. London: Royal Pharmaceutical Society of Great Britain and Merck Sharp and Dohme.

Royal College of Physicians (1990) *Research Involving Patients*. London: Royal College of Physicians.

Royal College of Physicians (1996). *Guidelines on the Practice of Ethics Committees in Medical Research Involving Human Subjects. Third edition*. London: Royal College of Physicians.

Royal Commission on the National Health Service (1979) *Report*. London: HMSO.

Royal Pharmaceutical Society of Great Britain (1997) *From Compliance to Concordance: Achieving Shared Goals in Medicine Taking*. London: Royal Pharmaceutical Society of Great Britain and Merck Sharp and Dohme.

Russell, L.B. (1986) *Is Prevention Better Than Cure?* Washington: Brookings Institution.

Ryan, J. with Thomas, F. (1997) *The Politics of Mental Handicap*. London: Free Association Books.

Saltman, R.B. and Otter, Von C. (1995) 'Vouchers in planned markets', in R.B. Saltman and Von C. Otter (eds), *Implementing Planned Markets in Health Care: Balancing Social and Economic Responsibility*. Buckingham: Open University Press.

Savulescu, J., Chalmers, I. and Blunt, J. (1996) 'Are research ethics committees behaving unethically? Some suggestions for improving performance', *British Medical Journal*, 313: 1390–3.

Schieber, G.J., Pouiller J-P. (1990). 'Overview of international comparisons of health care expenditures', in *Health Care Systems in Transition: The Search for Efficiency*. Paris: OECD.

Scott-Samuel. A. (ed.). (1990) *Total Participation, Total Health: Reinventing the Peckham Health Centre for the 1990s*. Edinburgh: Scottish Academic Press.

Senate of Surgery of Great Britain and Ireland (1997) *The Surgeon's Duty of Care*. London: Senate of Surgery of Great Britain and Ireland.

Shepperd, S., Coutler, A. and Farmer, A. (1995) 'Using interactive videos in general practice to inform patients about treatment choices: a pilot study', *Family Practice*, 12(4): 443–447.

Simpson, R. (1996) 'Relationship between self help health organisations and professional health care providers', *Health and Social Care in the Community*, 4 (6): 359–370.

Skrabanek, P. and McCormick, J. (1989) *Follies and Fallacies in Medicine*. Glasgow: Tarragon Press.

Skrzpiec, M. (1996) 'Work on patients' rights in Poland', in *Health Care in a Changing World: Patients' Rights and Responsibilities*. London: Consumers International and Slovene Consumers Association.

Sone, K. (1993) 'The visit', *Community Care*, 995: 18–19 (2 December).

Spiegal, D., Bloom, J. Kraemer, H.C. and Gottheil, E. (1989) 'Effect of psychosocial treatment on survival of patients with metastic breast cancer', *The Lancet*, 2 (ii): 888–891.

Spiers, H. (1998) 'Health service-speak is a foreign language to the public it serves', *Health Service Journal*, 12 February: 20.

Spiers, J. (1997) *Who Owns Our Bodies? Making Moral Choices in Health Care*. Oxford: Radcliffe Medical Press.

Stacey, M. (1992) *Regulating British Medicine: The General Medical Council*. Chichester: John Wiley and Sons.

Stewart, J., Kendall, E. and Coote, A. (1994) *Citizens' Juries*. London: Institute for Public Policy Research.

Stone, J. (1996) 'Beyond the fringe', *Health Matters*, 24: 18–19.

SW MIND (1996) *Avon Mental Health Measure*. Bristol: MIND.

Szaz, T.S. (1970) *The Manufacture of Madness*. London: Paladin.

Taylor, P. (1985) *The Smoke Ring: Tobacco, Money and Multinational Politics*, London: Bodley Head.

Thomas, D.H.V. and Noyce, P.R. (1996) 'The interface between self medication and the NHS', *British Medical Journal*, 312: 688–690.

Thomas, K., Fall, M., Parry, G. and Nicholl, J. (1995) *National Survey of Access to Complementary Health Care Via General Medical Practice*. Sheffield: Medical Care Research Unit, Sheffield Centre for Health and Related Research, Sheffield University.

Thompson, R. (1997) 'More patient choice?', *King's Fund News*, 20 (2): 4.

Thomson, W. (1992) 'Realising rights through local services'; in A. Coote (ed.), *The Welfare of Citizens: Developing New Social Rights*. London: Rivers Oram Press/Institute for Public Policy Research.

Titmuss, R.M. (1969). 'The culture of medical care and consumer behaviour', in F.N.L. Pynter (ed.), *Medicine and Culture*. Quoted in I. Illich (1975) *Medical Nemesis: The Expropriation of Health*. London: Calder and Boyars.

Tobias, J.S. (1997) 'BMJ's present policy (sometimes approving research in which patients have not given fully informed consent) is wholly correct', *British Medical Journal*, 314: 1111–14.

Tobias, S.J. and Souhami, R.L. (1993) 'Fully informed consent can be needlessly cruel', *British Medical Journal*, 307: 1199–1201.

Togerson, D. and Giuffrida, A. (1997) 'Paid to comply', *Health Service Journal*, 13 November: 30.

Townsend, P. and Davidson, N. (eds) (1988) *Inequalities in Health*. London: Penguin Books.

Tudor Hart, J. (1971) 'The inverse care law', *The Lancet*, 405–412.

Tudor Hart, J. (1994) *Feasible Socialism: the National Health Service Past Present and Future*. London: Socialist Health Association.

Turner, S., Longworth, A., Nunn, A.J. and Choonara, I. (1998) 'Unlicensed and off label drug use in paediatric wards', *British Medical Journal*: 316: 343–345.

Walker, M. (1993) *Dirty Medicine: Science, Big Business and the Assault on Natural Health Care*. London: Slingshot Publications.

Walt, G. (1993) 'WHO under stress: implications for health policy', *Health Policy*, 24: 125–144.

Watson, A. (1996) 'Generating problems? Power generation and health', in C. Hewett, C. Hogg, M. Leicester, and H. Rosenthal (eds), *Health and the Environment*. London: Socialist Health Association and the Socialist Environment and Resources Association.

Webster, C. (1996) 'Why has it taken so long to achieve so little?', *Health Matters*, 26: 5.

Webster, C. (1997) 'Eugenic sterilisation: Europe's shame', *Health Matters*, 31: 14–15.

Wenneras, C. and Wold, A. (1997) 'Nepotism and sexism in peer-review', *Nature*, 371 (6631): 341–343.

Westin, J.B. and Richter, E. (1990) 'The Israeli breast-cancer anomaly', Annals of the New York Academy of Sciences: 269–279. Quoted in S. Batt (1994) *Patient No More: The Politics of Breast Cancer*. London: Scarlet Press.

Whalley, T. and Barton, S. (1995) 'A purchaser perspective of managing new drugs: interferon beta as a case study', *British Medical Journal*, 311: 796–799.

WHO (1985) *Targets for Health For All*. Copenhagen: WHO Regional Office for Europe.

WHO (1990) *Environment and Health: The European Charter and Commentary*. Copenhagen: WHO Regional Office for Europe.

WHO (1994) *A Declaration on the Promotion of Patients' Rights in Europe*. Copenhagen: World Health Organization Regional Office for Europe.

WHO (1995) *Promotion of the Rights of Patients in Europe*. The Hague: Kluwer Law International.

Wilkinson, R. (1996) *Unhealthy Societies*. London: Routledge.

Williams, M.H. and Frankel, S.J. (1993). 'The myth of infinite demand', *Critical Public Health*, 4 (1): 13–17.

Williamson, C. (1992) *Whose Standards? Consumer and Professional Standards in Health Care*. Buckingham: Open University Press.

Williamson, C. (1995) 'A managers' guide to consumers', *Health Service Journal*, 30 November: 28–29.

Wilson, M. and Francis, J. (1997) *Raised Voices: African-Caribbean and African Users' Views and Experiences of Mental Health Services in England and Wales*. London: MIND.

Winslow, C., Kosecoff, J., Chassin, M., Kanouse, D. and Brook, H. (1988) 'The appropriateness of performing coronary artery bypass surgery', *Journal of the American Medical Association*, 260(4): 505–509.

Wise, J. (1997) 'Research suppressed for seven years by drug company', *British Medical Journal*, 314: 1145.

Wordsworth, S., Donaldson, C. and Scott, A. (1996) *Can We Afford the NHS?* London: Institute for Public Policy Research.

Wright, C.J. and Mueller, B. (1995) 'Screening mammography and public health policy: the need for perspective', *The Lancet*, 346: 29–31.

Yates, J. (1995) *Private Eye, Heart and Hip: Surgical Consultants, the National Health Service and Private Medicine.* Edinburgh: Churchill Livingstone.

INDEX

Access to Health Records Act 1990, 22
access to services, inequalities in,
23–27, 41, 48, 53, 62, 96, 120
accident and emergency services, 22
accountability, 108, 111, 173, 176–178;
of community health councils,
88–90; of family practitioners, 86–87;
of health authorities and trusts,
84–86; of lay representatives, 63
Action and Information on Sugars,
116, 154
Action for Sick Children, 42, 128, 130
adolescents, *see* children and young
people
advocacy, 25–27, 89, 90, 100,182
Age Concern, 130
Agenda 21, 107, 153
AIDS, *see* HIV/AIDS
alcohol, 20, 51, 62, 123; abuse of, 9, 27,
183; and health education, 52; and
pregnancy, 12
Alderson, Priscilla, 14
alternative therapies, *see*
complementary therapies
Alzheimer's disease, 31
American Medical International, 146
amniocentesis, 57
anorexia nervosa, 12, 13, 76, 183
antenatal care, 9, 26, 184; and drug
users, 24; and minority
communities, 26; and patient-held
records, 22; and screening, 56–57,
184; *see also* maternity services
antibiotics, 161, 162, 163
Armstrong, David, 63
Article 12, 132
Association for Improvements in the
Maternity Services (AIMS), 128, 131,
159, 184
Association for Public Health, 129

Association of Community Health
Councils for England and Wales, 25,
42, 88, 91, 135
Association of London Government,
107
Association of Medical Research
Charities, 71
Association of the British
Pharmaceutical Industry, 119
asthma, 40, 124, 126, 153, 166; research
on, 73; user centred services,
180–181
Attention deficit hyperactivity
disorders (ADHD), 12
Audit Commission, 30, 31, 41, 81, 91,
95
Australia, 118, 136–137, 177
Avon Mental Health Measure, 19
AZT (zidovudine), 66, 67, 74, 129

Baby Milk Action, 152
baby milk and infant foods, 151, 152,
154
Barham, Peter, 159, 182
Belgium, 54, 147
Bennet, Dr Glin, 29–30
benodiazepines, 78
Beresford, Peter, 26
beta interferon, 133, 167
Bevan, Aneurin, 85
Beveridge Report, 113
Bhatt, Sharon, 159
Black and Community Care Forum, 98
black and ethnic minority groups, 6,
25, 26, 59,148–149, 165, 182; access to
services, 23; and mental health
services, 8, 24, 93; and research
ethics committees, 69; user
involvement, 98, 108; and voluntary
sector, 93; *see also* refugees

Me

randomized controlled trials, 67–68; in screening programmes, 58–59; *see also* research ethics committees
ethnic minorities, people from, *see* black and ethnic minority groups
eugenics, 58–59
European Agency for the Evaluation of Medicinal Products (EMEA), 145
European Commission, 107, 140–141
European Patients Voice, 142
European Public Health Alliance, 140
European Union, 139–141, 147; and agriculture policy, 141, 153; and consumers, 140–143; and commercial interests, 152; and food safety, 154; and harmonization, 143–147; and health care market, 146; and pharmaceutical companies, 144–145; and public health, 149; and secrecy, 141
evidence-based medicine, 27, 160

family practitioners, 33; accountability of, 86–87, and complaints and discipline, 33–35; *see also* general practitioners
Faulder, Caroline, 11
Fernando, Suman, 24
Finland, 37, 54, 179
fluoridation, 62
focus groups, 75, 103
Food and Agriculture Organisation (FAO), 73, 139; and the Codex Alimentarius, 155–156
Food and Drug Administration (FAD), 73, 119
Food Commission, 156
food industry, 53; and government, 125–126; and international agencies, 154–156, *see also* baby milk and infant foods
Food Standards Agency, 116
FOREST (Freedom Organisation for the Right to Enjoy Smoking Tobacco), 124
France, 41, 60, 66, 110, 118, 143, 146, 170, 178
freedom of information, 30, 118–119; in Europe, 141, 177

Galton, Francis, 58
General Medical Council, 27–30, 35, 116, 134; case against Bristol cardiac surgeons, 29
general practitioners (GPs), 22, 23, 41, 45, 48, 85; accountability of, 86–87; and complaints procedures, 33–35; and complementary therapies, 39; and community health councils, 96, consultation by, 95–96; and immunization programmes, 60; and patients' charters, 44; and patient participation groups, 95; and pharmaceuticals, 41; and purchasing, 95, 121, 170; and research, 65; *see also* primary care
genetic testing, 57–59, 167
Germany, 41, 54, 55, 59, 99, 143, 153
Gillick, Victoria, 15
Glasgow, 106
Goodare, Heather, 185
government departments, 112–115; advisory committees of, 116–118; and commercial interests, 113, 122–126; and professional interests, 121–122
Greece, 54, 118
Green, David, 28
Griffiths Report (NHS Management Inquiry), 165
Griffiths, Sir Roy, 94

Harris, John, 37
Health Action International, 40, 142, 144, 145, 151
health authorities, 31, 38, 108, 116, 121, 133, 170; and accountability, 86; and community health councils, 90–91; and complementary therapies, 39; and consultation, 94–96; and continuing care, 120; and Health of the Nation, 52; and local authorities, 85; and locality commissioning, 95–97; and needs assessment, 96, 102–105; and rationing, 97–99, 169; and research ethics committees, 68, 70; and the voluntary sector, 92–93
Health Education Authority, 107
health education, *see* health promotion
health gain, 98, 161